DISCLAIMERS

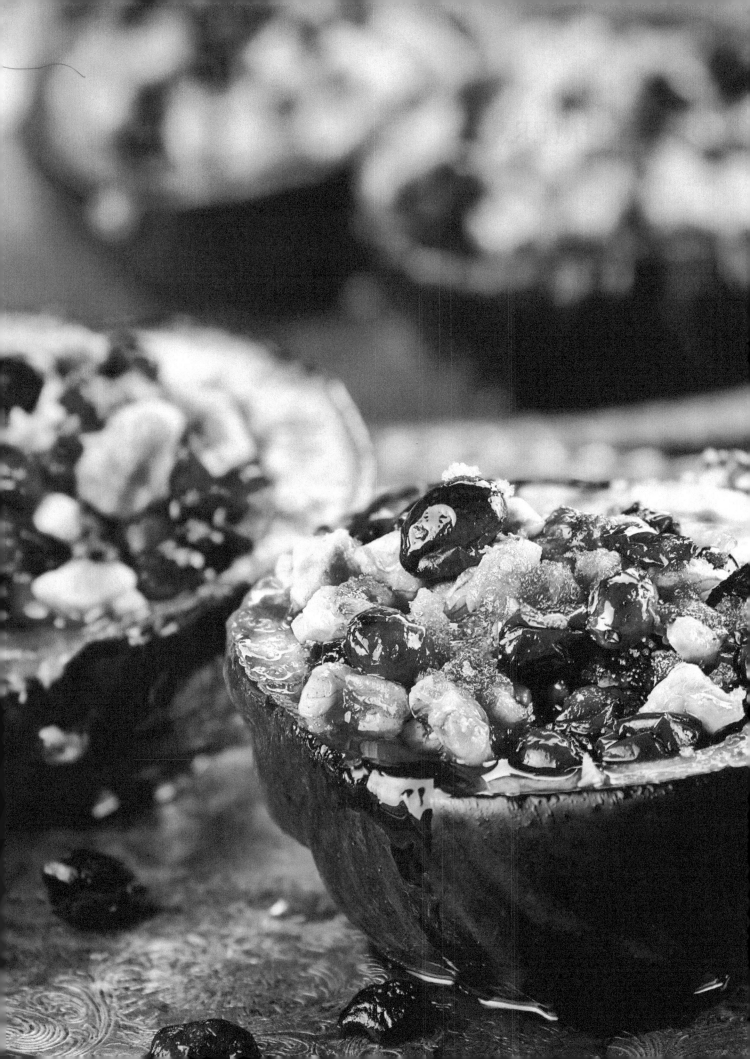

WELCOME

Hello and welcome! I'm so excited you are here and taking this step to improve your health. I am honored that you have allowed me to be a part of your journey.

By the age of 25, I was diagnosed with high blood sugar, chronic fatigue syndrome, fibromyalgia, and depression. I was also carrying an extra 20 pounds, and I felt tired, frustrated, and defeated. I knew food played a significant role in these conditions and in causing inflammation, but I tried diet after diet with no success.

I made every mistake the first time around...eating too many or too few calories in a day, only focusing on the number on the scale, and jumping on the latest fad diet in the hopes that this time it would finally work and I would feel better.

From yo-yo dieting to sustainable healthy habits in just a few weeks...
I completely abandoned my previous beliefs about health and weight loss and took a deep dive into all the research available to me. Known as one of the healthiest diets in the world, the Mediterranean diet is often recommended for long-term health and disease prevention, and it consistently showed up in my research findings. I started to follow a low-carb Mediterranean-based diet, and within the first week, I had lost 4 pounds! I went on to lose a total of 20 pounds over the next 3 months and drastically improve my overall quality of health, including **completely reversing my chronic fatigue, fibromyalgia, and depression and lowering my blood sugar.**

I was so ecstatic about my results that I put together all the recipes I had developed during this time and started sharing them with others, hoping they would feel just as amazing as I felt. In this book, I have included all that I have learned and all the tools I used on my health journey. I hope that you find incredible value in this book, and I am so excited for you to experience the same results.

In health,

Rachel, founder of Beyond the Brambleberry
www.beyondthebrambleberry.com

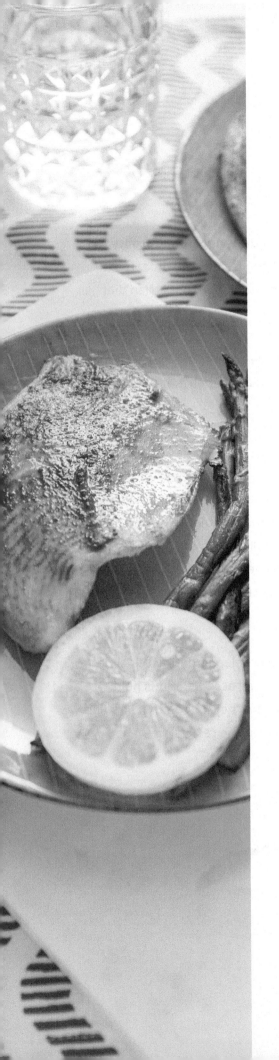

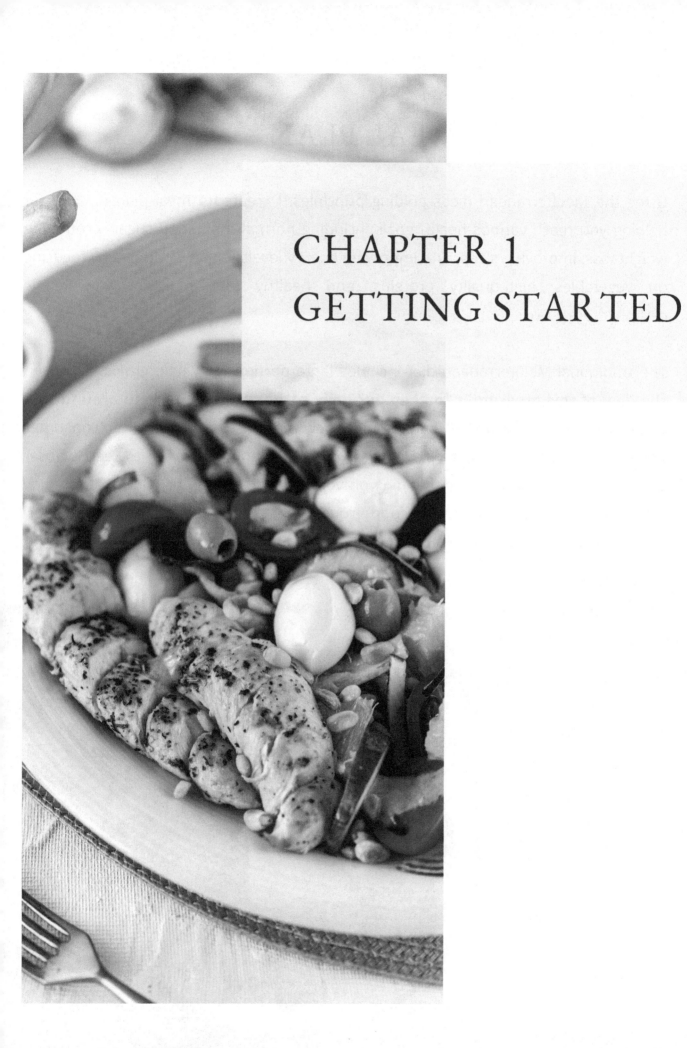

CHAPTER 1
GETTING STARTED

ABOUT THIS MEAL PLAN

Using the Mediterranean diet's guiding principles, I created a meal plan optimal for helping you reach various health goals including normalizing blood sugar, promoting weight loss, improving sleep, and improving energy levels. I have done this by focusing on vegetables, high-quality proteins, and healthy fats and closely watching carbohydrate intake.

The traditional Mediterranean diet includes large portions of whole grains. However, **the goal of this program is to keep our daily carbohydrate intake to around 25% of our daily consumption of food**. Studies show that the average American consumes between 250-300 grams of carbs every day. Our goal in this program is to keep it closer to 100-150 grams each day, depending on your caloric needs. This allows us to enjoy more foods from other nutritious food groups and to promote health without over-restricting one specific food group.

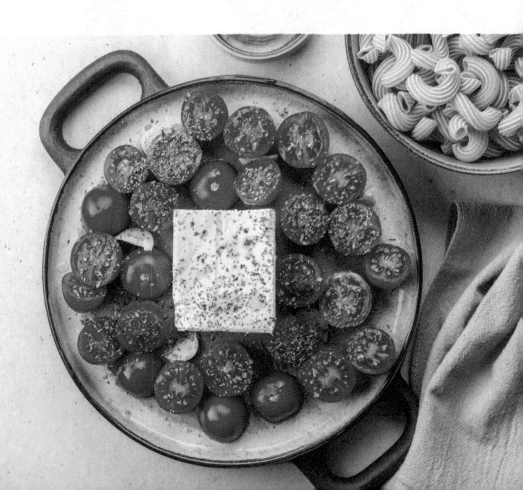

As I mentioned before, this is the exact meal plan that I used to lose 20 pounds and reverse several health conditions. That being said, I want to highlight a few key points:

- I have a gluten intolerance and do not consume any gluten. Therefore, all of these recipes are gluten-free or have gluten-free options. If you do not follow a gluten-free diet, you can absolutely still enjoy these recipes and follow this meal plan. You may even discover that you feel better not eating as much gluten as it is inflammatory for many people.
- I am also lactose intolerant (lucky me), but I am able to tolerate cheese made from sheep and goat milk. I am also able to tolerate some cow's milk products each day by taking a daily probiotic. Dairy is limited in this program, but when I do incorporate it into my diet, I consume high-quality cheeses and Greek yogurt. Give these recipes a try and see if you notice a difference in how your gut feels when you don't include as much dairy in your diet. I am also convinced that taking out these gut-irritating foods is what contributed to my weight loss success and overall improvement in health.

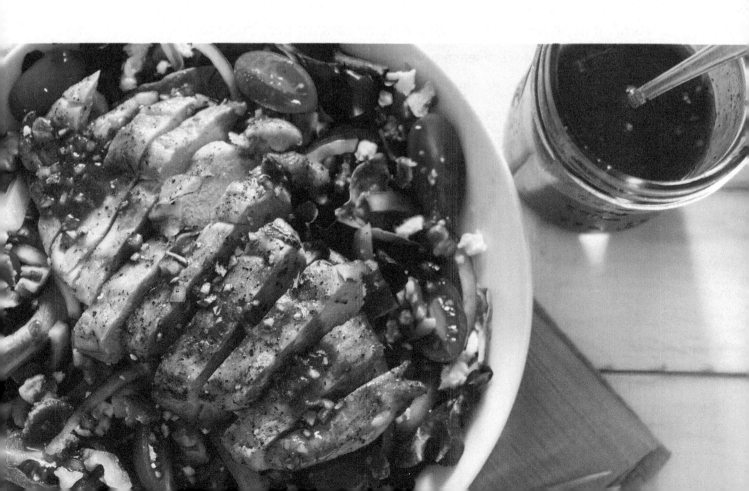

THE MEDITERRANEAN DIET

What is the Mediterranean diet?

The Mediterranean Diet is a diet that focuses on eating lots of healthy fats, whole grains, fruits, vegetables, nuts, seeds, beans, and legumes. It became popular in the 1950s when it was discovered that people living in the Mediterranean region had a drastically lower rate of heart disease. Many studies have been done on this diet since that time and have shown that the Mediterranean diet provides many health benefits.

The Mediterranean diet focuses on:
- Healthy fats rich in Omega-3s
- Eating fish at least twice a week
- Preparing meals with lots of vegetables, served with whole grains and high-quality protein
- Enjoying lots of fresh fruit, especially for dessert

Potential health benefits of the Mediterranean diet include:
- Lower risk of heart disease and stroke
- Lower risk of obesity, high cholesterol, diabetes, and high blood pressure
- Support in weight loss and sustaining a healthy weight
- Promotion of longevity
- Improved brain health and decreased risk of developing dementia

Eating red meat on the Mediterranean diet

Red meat is a controversial subject in the nutrition world, but recent studies have shown the health benefits of incorporating unprocessed red meat into a balanced diet. As red meat is high in important vitamins and minerals including zinc, iron, and B vitamins, I incorporate it into this meal plan. If you are trying to cut down on the amount of red meat you consume, you can easily replace it with other protein sources in these recipes. For example, ground beef can easily be replaced with ground turkey or chicken.

How to follow the Mediterranean diet when you don't live in the Mediterranean.
The goal of this meal plan is to help you follow a Mediterranean-based diet that is realistic for where you live. As most of us do not live in the Mediterranean region, I created recipes that are affordable and that include ingredients that are easily accessible. Therefore, the recipes in this meal plan focus on the principles of the Mediterranean diet including eating lots of fruits, vegetables, healthy fats, unprocessed lean proteins, beans, legumes, and whole grains in moderation.

••

If you are interested in diving more into the research of the many health benefits of the Mediterranean diet, check out these links:

- **Mediterranean Diet for Heart Health**: https://www.mayoclinic.org/healthy-lifestyle/nutrition-and-healthy-eating/in-depth/mediterranean-diet/art-20047801
- **American Heart Association: What Is The Mediterranean Diet?**: https://www.heart.org/en/healthy-living/healthy-eating/eat-smart/nutrition-basics/mediterranean-diet
- **A Mediterranean-style eating pattern with lean, unprocessed red meat has cardiometabolic benefits for adults who are overweight or obese in a randomized, crossover, controlled feeding trial:** https://www.ncbi.nlm.nih.gov/pmc/articles/PMC6600057/

GUIDELINES

There are rules?! Well, really more like "guidelines." The guidelines outlined below will put you on the fast track toward creating sustainable habits that will support you in reaching your health goals.

Use healthy fats and oils for cooking

Extra virgin olive oil and avocado oil are the oils I use the most as they are filled with healthy omega-3 fats. Many of your healthy fats will also come from the high-quality meats you consume in this meal plan. Other sources of fat will include high-quality cheeses (especially feta and goat cheese), nuts, and seeds.

Invest in high-quality proteins

Choosing the right proteins to purchase and consume means the difference between eating beef that was kept in a stall and fed corn for its entire life (something that is not natural for a cow) versus eating beef that was able to roam the pastures and eat grass all day (the makings for a very happy cow). The same goes for any type of meat you buy. Animals should be living as close to their natural lives as possible to provide the most nutritious meat.

Look for the following labels when grocery shopping:

- Pasture-raised eggs
- Free range chicken
- Grass-fed, grass-finished beef, bison, etc.

These sources of protein are a little more costly, but remember, you get what you pay for. Invest in yourself and put in your body the very best that is possible. You deserve it.

Choose your carbs wisely

I am not a fan of extremely restrictive diets. While this diet may seem restrictive to some at first, once you get into the swing of it, you will realize just how many options you have for meals. However, one thing we must be mindful of is our carbohydrate consumption. The average American consumes between 250-300 grams (or more) of carbohydrates every day. Here, our goal is closer to 100-150 grams per day.

Do not get me wrong... healthy carbs are part of a well-balanced diet. That being said, it is important to choose the right carbohydrates to eat so that you are getting the most bang for your buck nutritionally.

When you are choosing carbohydrates, consider these healthy options:
- Quinoa
- Red potatoes
- Sweet potatoes
- Brown rice
- Jasmine rice
- Oats
- Beans
- Legumes

Also, as a general rule, I choose one meal each day to get my "carb fix." For me, I usually choose one of the following for the day:
- a waffle or piece of toast for breakfast (both gluten free)
- a roasted sweet potato or squash in my salad for lunch, OR
- a potato, beans, or legumes with dinner

Fall in love with leftovers and meal-prepping

If you are one of those people who hates leftovers, you will be doing a lot more cooking every day. Making enough food for leftovers makes this meal plan a thousand times easier to stick with and will drastically decrease the time you spend in the kitchen cooking. Instead, cook once, and eat for days!

Find a few healthy meals you love and make them on repeat

I have talked to many healthy living practitioners, and one thing they all do (including myself) is stick to a handful of healthy recipes that they love and put them on their rotation for regular meal planning. By doing this, you become extremely efficient in making these meals and will most likely have the ingredients on hand or on your upcoming shopping list. If you find you have a little extra time in one week, choose a new recipe to try to potentially add to your rotation.

Stop eating 2-3 hours before you go to bed

This gives your body time to digest the food you have eaten and for blood sugar levels to return to normal before your body goes into "rest and digest" mode.

Your daily meal plan should look something like this:
- A high-protein and high-fat breakfast
- A large salad for lunch
- A handful of nuts with fruit for a snack
- A dinner with protein and lots of vegetables several hours before bed

Eat at least 1,200 calories every day (preferably 1,400 calories or more)

You must eat **at least** 1,200 calories every single day in order to give your body the macronutrients and micronutrients it needs to thrive. I personally do not recommend eating less than 1,400 calories, but I know some people might resist that. But please, do not restrict yourself more than this. Your body needs fuel and nourishment to function at its best, and severe calorie restriction will not help you reach your health goals any faster.

Enjoy fruit, but don't overindulge

Fruit is often higher in sugar, and while this sugar is accompanied by lots of healthy fiber, vitamins, and antioxidants, it can affect your blood sugar and weight loss efforts. Try to stick to only a few servings of fruit each day, and choose lower-sugar fruits such as berries.

Engage in exercise at least 3 days a week

I have never been an overly athletic person. There was a six-month window where I was going to the gym nearly every day, but that came to a grinding halt when my husband and I took a one-month trip home to visit family and I never returned to my workout routine. I had always believed my workout routines had to kick my butt and make it difficult to get out of bed the next morning. However, finding an activity you enjoy doing regularly is the key to keeping active.

I personally enjoy yoga, walking, and dumbbell workouts. Over the last year, I have stepped up my yoga flows to include more strength and bodyweight training, however, I started gently and developed a practice I enjoyed. If you are interested in starting a yoga practice at home, I highly recommend checking out **Breathe and Flow** or **Cat Meffan** on YouTube. I absolutely love their yoga flows and got into incredible physical shape with their videos - all from my living room for free!

Other exercises you may be interested in exploring include:
- walking or hiking
- bicycling
- bodyweight training
- dumbbell exercises
- dancing
- tai chi
- barre
- rock climbing
- rebounding

COMMON QUESTIONS

Fresh vs. canned vs. frozen: which is better?

I believe fresh produce is always the best choice. My second choice is frozen because the vegetables are frozen at the time of their peak nutritional value. If you are going to buy canned, look for "BPA-free" labels.

Why is there not a lot of dairy and cheese included in these recipes?

In my introduction, I explained that I am sharing the exact recipes and meal plan I used to lose 20 pounds in 3 months and drastically improve my health. For me, cutting out dairy was a necessity to feel my best as I am lactose intolerant. I am able to ingest dairy with the daily use of a probiotic, so I do incorporate some dairy into my meals. While many people are not lactose intolerant, I believe it would benefit many people to try to eat dairy-free for a time (or at least decrease the amount of dairy they consume) to see if they feel a difference. Lactose sensitivity can be sneaky and hard to identify, so why not enjoy these delicious, dairy-free recipes and see if you experience less bloating, less gas, and clearer skin? You may be surprised by the results.

I do include grass-fed butter, ghee, feta cheese, and goat cheese in my recipes because I personally do not experience adverse symptoms as long as I take a probiotic. If you are lactose intolerant and find that you cannot tolerate butter, I recommend trying ghee or olive oil in its place.

Why am I not losing weight on the Mediterranean diet?

If your goal is to lose weight by following this meal plan, be mindful of the following factors that can interfere with you reaching your goals.

- **Hidden food sensitivities:** gluten and dairy sensitivities are the most common, and these can stall your weight loss progress. Your body does not want to focus on weight loss if it is inflamed and irritated by food sensitivities. If you aren't getting the results you want, try cutting out gluten and dairy from your meals for a while and see how you feel.

- **Too many carbs or fruit:** You can have too much of a good thing, and in a weight loss journey, carbs and fruit can stall your progress. Keep a close eye on how many carbs you are eating each day. In this program, we try to keep our carb count between 100-150 grams every day.

- **Too many nuts (too much fat):** While extremely nutrient-dense, nuts are higher in calories and fat. This is another example of having too much of a good thing. Try to enjoy around ¼ cup of nuts each day.

- **Not eating enough:** As you count calories, are you finding that you are not reaching your daily caloric intake goal? Our bodies go into "storage mode" when we do not eat enough. If you find you are not eating enough calories, try eating an additional serving or two of nuts or nut butter.

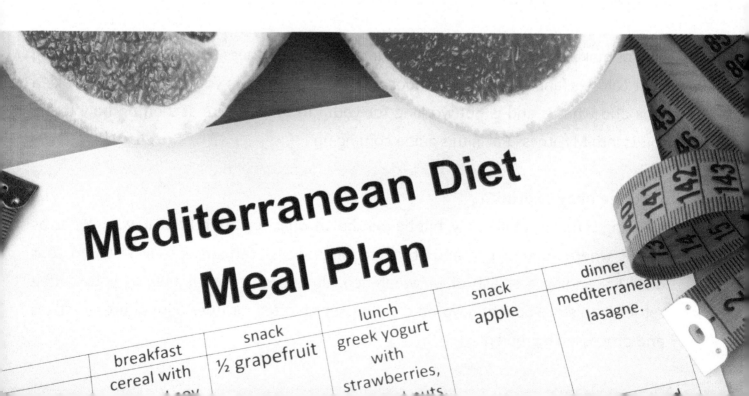

Can I substitute ingredients in these recipes?

It depends. You can certainly substitute different meats and vegetables in these recipes. Using ground turkey instead of ground beef because that is what you have on hand is 100% okay. Additionally, if a recipe calls for almond milk and you want to use cow's milk, it's not the end of the world. However, I would like to remind you of what I mentioned in the previous section regarding giving dairy free recipes a try to see if you feel a difference in your health.

Should I be counting calories?

In this meal plan, we do count calories, and I believe it is extremely helpful in any weight loss journey. I personally count calories each day and believe it is beneficial to do so at least for a time as it helps you get an idea of how many calories are really in your food. If you decide later to stop counting calories, you will at least have a basic idea of how many calories you are eating each day and will be more mindful of your choices.

If you take one thing away from this section, let it be this: **not all calories are created equal**. Your body does not process 160 calories of peanut butter cups the same way it does 160 calories of grass-fed beef or raw cashews. This is why we not only count calories but create nourishing meals made with whole foods.

Do not make counting calories a difficult task. Use MyFitness Pal or a similar app to log your calories (and weight if you choose). It's free and allows you to go back and take a look and what is and is not working for you. I have an entire section on how to log foods into MyFitness Pal in this guide coming up.

Is coffee okay to drink?

Drinking coffee is totally okay, but be mindful of what you are putting in your coffee as that is where added sugar and processed ingredients can sneak their way into your diet. Try adding a splash of unsweetened almond or coconut milk to your coffee rather than store-bought flavored creamer, which often includes a lot of preservatives and processed ingredients.

COUNTING CALORIES AND KEEPING A FOOD LOG

Counting calories is a topic often debated in the health industry. Some people swear by it, while others say you should not count calories and should instead eat intuitively. I personally see value in counting calories, especially when trying to lose weight. However, it is only one of several tools I use to maintain a healthy lifestyle. I am a fan of counting calories and believe it is beneficial to do so, at least for a time, as it helps you get an idea of how many calories you are generally consuming each day. If you later decide to stop counting calories, you will at least have a basic idea of how many calories your food contains.

It is also easy to enjoy too much of a good thing. For example, while cashews are highly nutritious, they are higher in calories and can be easy to overeat. This is why we measure out only ¼ cup of cashews and log them in our food journal to ensure we are eating a balanced diet.

Do not make counting calories a difficult thing. I recommend using MyFitness Pal or a similar app to log your calories (and weight if you choose). It's free and allows you to go back and take a look and what is and is not working for you. If you do not want to log your food online, keeping a paper journal works just as well. I provide the calorie, carb, protein, and fat counts for all of the recipes shared here. The big thing to focus on is the total calorie count. Your protein, carb, fat, and sugar intake will fluctuate each day, and you will drive yourself crazy if you try to keep it perfectly balanced every day (speaking from experience).

Let's get started!

CALCULATE YOUR CALORIC NEEDS

Step 1: Go to the macro calculator by going to:

http://www.jameslaytonfitnessinnercircle.com/iifym-calculator/index.html

Step 2: Fill in the information in the first section. **BE HONEST** with the information. "Stretching the truth" will only sabotage your health goals. If you are currently a couch potato, check off that you are a couch potato! If you don't know your current body fat %, that's okay - just leave it blank.

Calorie and macro nutrient calculator

GENDER	AGE	HEIGHT	WEIGHT
○ MALE ◉ FEMALE	26 YEARS	5 FT 2 IN	124 LBS

◉ IMPERIAL ○ METRIC

FORMULA
◉ ATHLETES FORMULA (BEST FOR LEAN PEOPLE)
○ LEAN MASS FORMULA (BEST IF OVERWEIGHT)

EXERCISE LEVEL
3 times/week

CURRENT BODY FAT %

YOUR BMR IS: 1257 CALORIES/DAY

YOUR TDEE IS: 1728 CALORIES/DAY

CALCULATE YOUR TDEE

Step 3: Click the red **"Calculate your TDEE."**

Your BMR is your Basal Metabolic Rate. This is the absolute **fewest** number of calories your body needs each day to perform all its necessary tasks (i.e. brain function, heart function, digestion, etc.)

Your TDEE is your Total Daily Energy Expenditure. These additional calories allow you to perform the exercises and additional activities you do in a day. This number is the number you want to focus on when trying to **maintain** weight.

Step 4: Scroll down to the next section. You can play around with this section to see how the numbers change, but in this guide, we are going to use the **suggested 15% weight loss** button. This is what I did and still lost 20 lbs in 3 months!

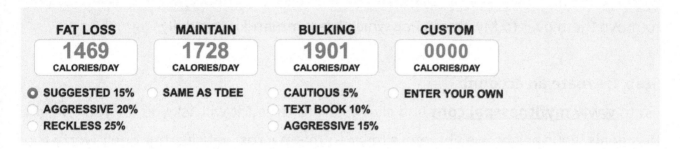

Step 5: Scroll down to the next section and click "Low Carb" under "Common Plans."

Step 6: Adjust the Fat, Carbs & Protein percentages to read: **Fat 50%, Carbs 25%, Proteins 25%**. Then click "Calculate." Your results will generate below.

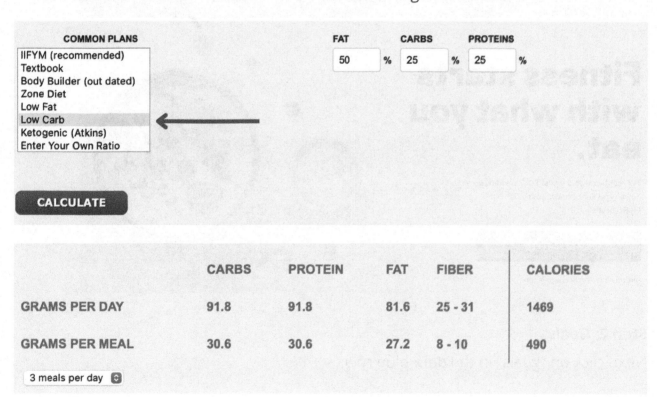

	CARBS	PROTEIN	FAT	FIBER	CALORIES
GRAMS PER DAY	91.8	91.8	81.6	25 - 31	1469
GRAMS PER MEAL	30.6	30.6	27.2	8 - 10	490

3 meals per day

COPYING MACROS TO MYFITNESS PAL

Now that we have our calorie, protein, carbohydrate, and fat goals calculated, it's time to move them over to MyFitness Pal, which I recommend using daily.

Step 1: Create an account

Go to **www.myfitnesspal.com** and click "Start for free." It will ask you for your weight loss goals, your height, weight, etc. similar to the macros website, but don't worry too much about that and the results it gives you. Just go through the steps to create an account, and we will adjust everything once we are logged in.

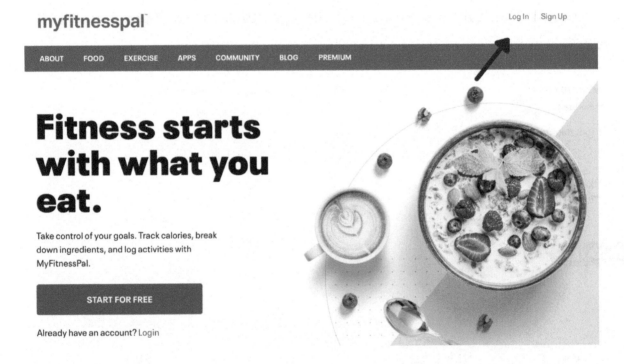

Step 2: Goals

Next, click on "goals" in the dark blue row.

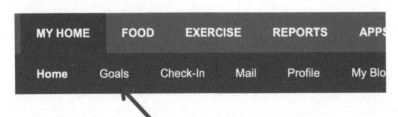

Step 3: Daily Nutrition Goals

Click "Edit" under Daily Nutrition Goals.

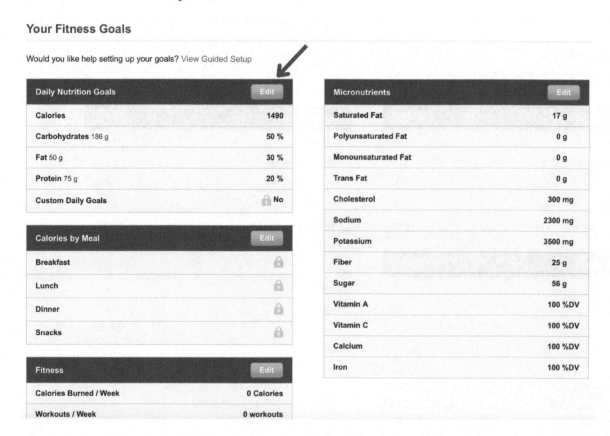

Adjust your calorie and macronutrient goals according to what we calculated from the macronutrient calculator in the previous section: **Custom Calories, Fat 50%, Carbs 25%, Protein 25%**. Click "Save Changes" when you are done.

Daily Nutrition Goals

Calories		1469
Macronutrients		🔒 Set by Grams
Carbohydrates 92 g		25% ↕
Fat 82 g		50% ↕
Protein 92 g		25% ↕
% Total Macronutrients must equal 100%		100%

Step 4: Set Your Sugar Goal

The last thing to change is your sugar goal.

Click on "Edit" under the micronutrients tab and change your daily sugar goal to **45 g**.

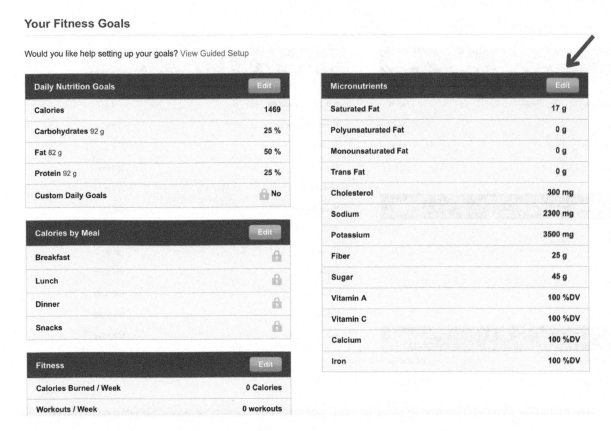

Step 5: Start Logging

You are all set! Now, when you click the "Food" Tab to view your Food Diary, your daily goals will be outlined for you.

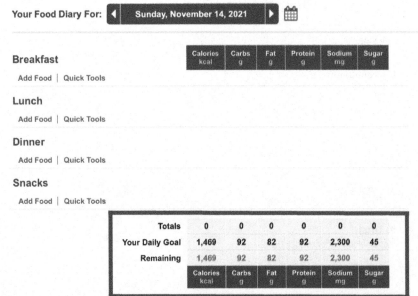

ESTABLISH HEALTHY ROUTINES

01

Get at least 7 hours of sleep every night.

Your body does so much for you while you are sleeping including detoxifying, strengthening your immune system, and repairing muscle. Make it a priority to get at least 7 hours of sleep every night to give your body enough time to do its reparative work.

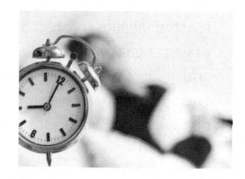

02

Eat a filling breakfast with protein and healthy fat.

I believe breakfast is the most important meal of the day. If I don't eat a breakfast full of protein and healthy fat, my whole day will feel "off" and I will feel especially hungry the rest of the day. Occasionally I will add a healthy carb (such as low-carb waffles or a piece of whole-grain toast with ghee) to help keep me fuller for longer.

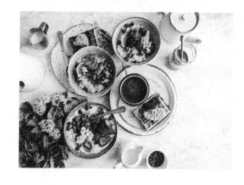

03

Eat a lunch full of veggies and healthy protein.

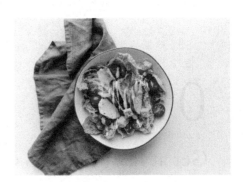

I love making big salads for lunch with lots of roasted veggies, protein such as baked chicken thighs, healthy additions including nuts, feta, and goat cheese, and a homemade dressing. The possibilities are endless, and you will discover some delicious recipes through this meal plan.

04

Keep healthy snacks on hand.

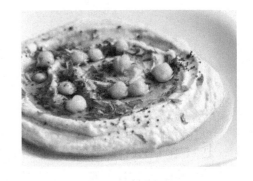

If you need a snack between meals, be sure to choose healthy options and log them into MyFitness Pal to make sure you don't go over your daily caloric needs. If you find yourself needing frequent snacks throughout the day, take a look at your meals and consider if they include enough protein and healthy fat to keep you full until the next meal. You may need to eat slightly larger meals to prevent hunger between meals.

05

Eat dinner 2-3 hours before bed.

Dinner in this meal plan typically consists of healthy protein and vegetables cooked in liberal amounts of olive oil, avocado oil, or ghee. Try to eat dinner 2-3 hours before bed to give your body time to digest before you lay down. I sometimes add a healthy carbohydrate to this meal such as a red potato or sweet potato.

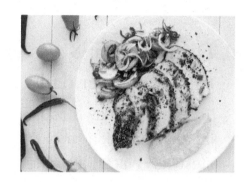

06

Engage in 30 minutes of physical activity at least 3 days a week.

Physical activity is so important in maintaining a healthy weight, promoting good circulation and digestion, aiding in restful sleep, and so much more. You don't have to do anything too intense, but find some sort of movement that you enjoy. Examples include walking, yoga, dance, bicycling, and bodyweight exercises.

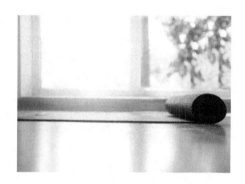

07

Drink at least 8 glasses (64 ounces total) of water daily.

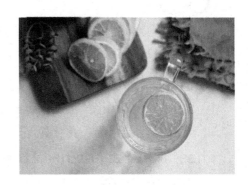

The human body is roughly 60% water, making its consumption a vital part of a healthy lifestyle. Water also helps promote healthy digestion, supports heart and lung function, cushions the brain, and supports healthy hormone function.

MEDITERRANEAN SHOPPING LIST

VEGETABLES

- acorn squash
- artichoke
- asparagus
- beets
- bell peppers
- broccoli
- brussels sprouts
- butternut squash
- cabbage
- carrots
- cauliflower
- celery
- chard
- corn
- cucumber
- eggplant
- greens - arugula, lettuce, spinach, collards, kale, alfalfa, etc.
- green beans
- leeks
- mushrooms
- okra
- olives
- onion - red, yellow, green
- peas
- pumpkin
- radishes
- scallions
- spaghetti squash
- summer squash
- tomatoes
- turnips
- zucchini

FRUIT

- apples
- apricots
- bananas
- berries - strawberries, blackberries, raspberries, blueberries
- cherries
- clementines
- figs
- grapefruit
- grapes
- kiwi
- lemons
- limes
- mangoes
- medjool dates
- melons - watermelon, cantaloupe, honeydew, etc.
- nectarines
- olives
- oranges
- peaches
- pears
- pineapple
- plums
- pomegranate
- rhubarb
- strawberries

MEDITERRANEAN SHOPPING LIST

MEAT & FISH

- chicken
- fish - tuna, salmon, trout, halibut, cod, shrimp, lobster, scallops, crab, sardines, etc.
- grass-fed beef (around 80% lean)
- lamb
- organ meats - heart, liver, etc.
- pork, ham, bacon (nitrate-free preferably), sausage
- turkey
- venison

HEALTHY FATS

- avocado
- avocado oil
- coconut milk and coconut cream
- coconut oil
- extra virgin olive oil
- grass-fed butter
- grass-fed ghee

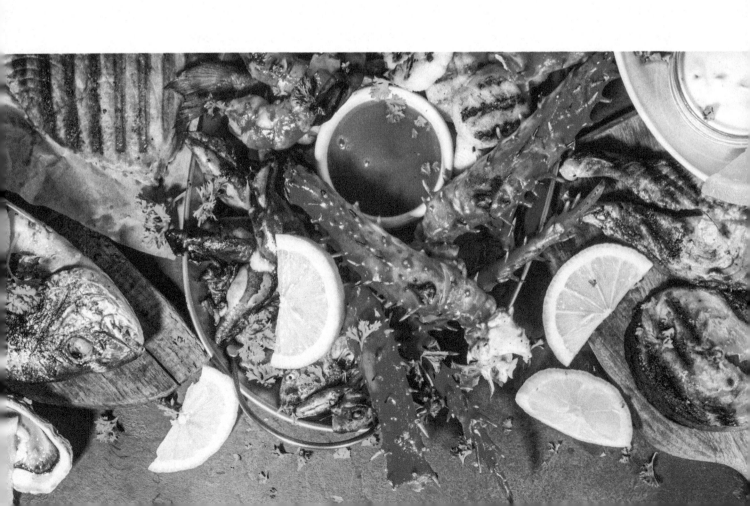

MEDITERRANEAN SHOPPING LIST

DAIRY & EGGS

- feta cheese
- goat cheese
- grass-fed butter
- ghee (usually found in the olive oil and spices section of the grocery store)
- Greek yogurt (whole, plain)
- pasture-raised eggs

SPICES, HERBS, & PANTRY STAPLES

- basil
- cilantro
- cinnamon
- cloves
- coriander
- cumin
- fennel
- garlic
- ginger
- Italian seasoning
- mint
- nutmeg
- oregano
- parsley
- red pepper flake
- rosemary
- thyme
- vanilla
- vinegar - balsamic, white, white wine, red wine, apple cider

WHOLE GRAINS & CARBS

- beans: kidney, black, chickpea (garbanzo), cannellini (white), pinto, fava, etc.
- barley
- bulgur
- bread (preferably whole-grain)
- couscous
- hummus
- lentils
- oatmeal
- pasta - preferably whole-grain
- polenta
- quinoa
- red potatoes
- rice
- sweet potatoes

HEALTHY SWEETENERS

- honey (local if possible)
- maple syrup (local if possible)
- molasses
- monkfruit powder
- stevia

MEDITERRANEAN SHOPPING LIST

NUTS & SEEDS

- almonds & almond butter
- cashews & cashew butter
- chia seeds
- edamame
- hazelnuts
- macadamia nuts
- peanuts & peanut butter
- pecans
- pine nuts
- pistachios
- pumpkin seeds (pepitas)
- sesame seeds
- sunflower seeds
- walnuts

Look for raw or dry roasted nuts.

BEVERAGES

- bone broth
- coffee
- seltzer water & club soda (zero sugar)
- tea
- water
- wine (in moderation)

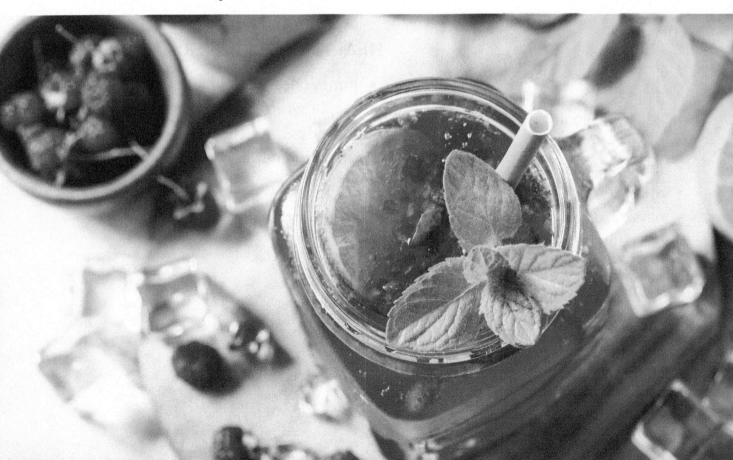

RECOMMENDED PRODUCTS

There are a few products I buy to step up my health food game, and I am sharing them here as I reference some of them in the upcoming recipes. I use these products specifically because they are lower in sugar, made with whole foods, and have supported me in reaching my health goals. You can find many of these foods at your local grocery store, but you can also find links to purchasing them online on Beyond the Brambleberry's online shop at
https://www.beyondthebrambleberry.com/resource-page.

- King Arthur's Measure for Measure Gluten-Free Flour
- Birch Benders' Paleo Pancake & Waffle Mix
- Cup4Cup Gluten Free Flour
- Primal Kitchen Ketchup
- Primal Kitchen BBQ Sauce
- Primal Kitchen Alfredo Sauce
- Rao's Marinara Sauce
- Siete Red Enchilada Sauce

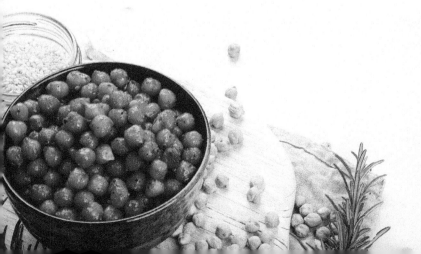

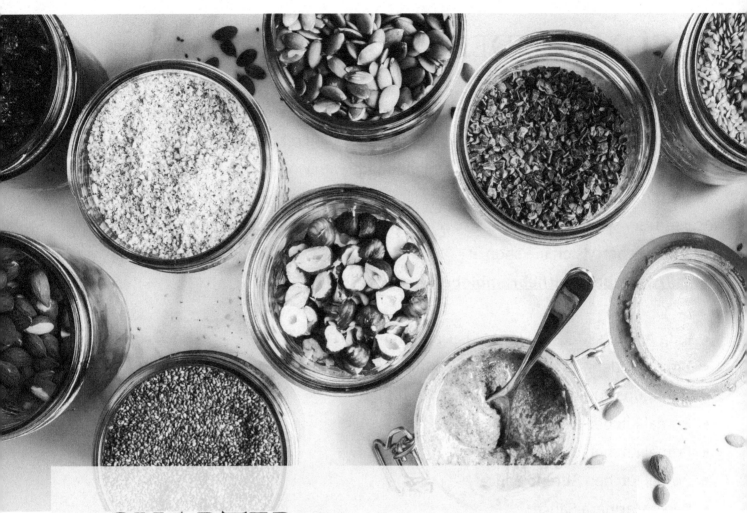

CHAPTER 2
PANTRY STAPLES, SEASONINGS, DIPS & SAUCES

PANTRY & KITCHEN STAPLES

Premade seasonings

Store-bought seasonings often contain high amounts of salt and preservatives. Making your own seasonings is easy and avoids the unhealthy ingredients found in store-bought products. Check out the recipes provided in this meal plan to get started.

Raw nuts and seeds

Raw nuts and seeds are a great addition to the pantry as they are so versatile to use in recipes. They make great snacks, are delicious additions to salads, and are high in healthy fats. Just be sure to purchase raw nuts and seeds and not roasted as these often contain unhealthy oils, sugars, and salt. If you want roasted nuts, roast them at home or purchase them dry-roasted.

Chia seeds

Chia seeds provide a quick and easy snack option (such as in chia pudding) and provide a ton of fiber, protein, and calcium in one serving. A great chia pudding recipe is included in this meal plan.

Olive and avocado oil

Olive oil and avocado oil are what we use most in this guide, and they are both high-quality choices of fat. They are great options for stovetop cooking and for roasting in the oven.

Vinegar: balsamic, white, and apple cider vinegar

In combination with olive and avocado oil, these vinegars make the base for delicious dressings. Pick up a bottle of each at the store and be prepared for an endless variety of salad dressings.

TACO SEASONING

INGREDIENTS

- 2 Tablespoons chili powder
- ½ teaspoon garlic powder
- ½ teaspoon onion powder
- ½ teaspoon red pepper flakes
- ½ teaspoon dried oregano
- 1 teaspoon dried paprika
- 1 teaspoon cumin
- 2 teaspoons salt
- 2 teaspoons black pepper

DIRECTIONS

1. Combine all ingredients in a mason jar.
2. Use 1-2 Tablespoons for every 1 pound of ground meat, depending on personal preference.

NOTES

- Use this seasoning with ground beef, turkey, or chicken to make delicious burrito bowls, or rub onto chicken breasts and thighs.

FAJITA SEASONING

INGREDIENTS

- 1 Tablespoon chili powder
- 2 teaspoons dried paprika
- ½ teaspoon garlic powder
- ½ teaspoon onion powder
- ½ teaspoon red pepper flakes
- ½ teaspoon dried oregano
- ½ teaspoon cumin
- 2 teaspoons cayenne pepper
- 2 teaspoons salt
- 2 teaspoons black pepper

DIRECTIONS

1. Combine all ingredients in a mason jar.
2. Use 1-2 Tablespoons for every 1 pound of ground meat, depending on personal preference.

NOTES

- Use with ground beef, turkey, or chicken to make delicious fajita stir-fries, or rub on chicken breasts and thighs.

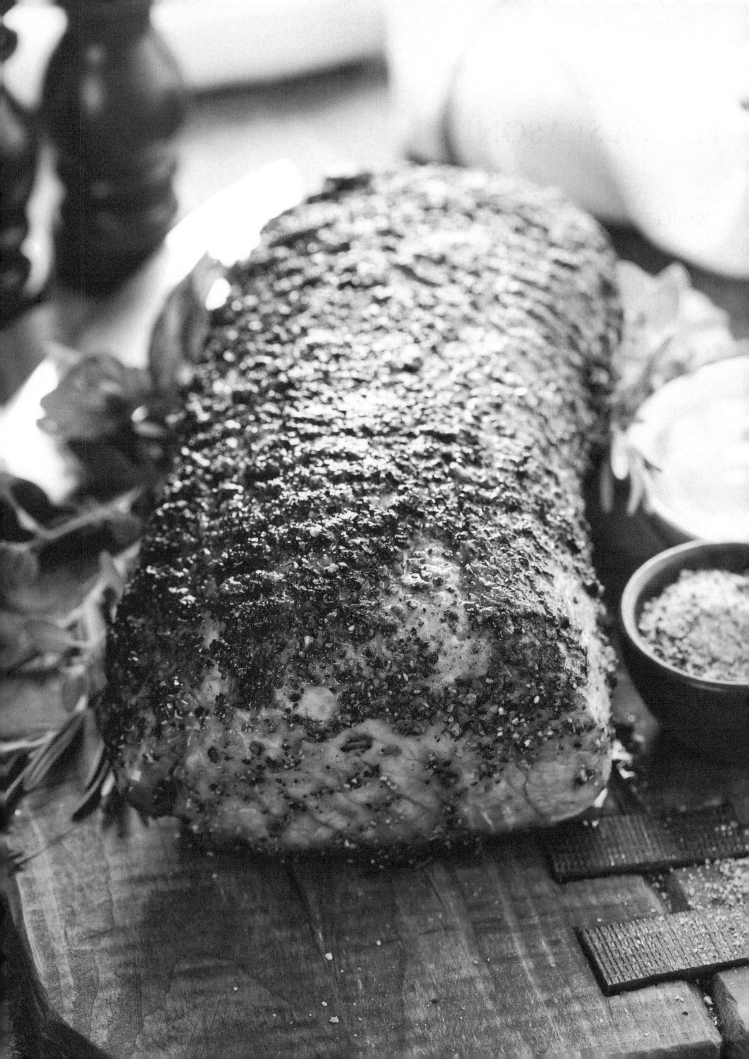

THE BEST PORK RUB

INGREDIENTS

- ¼ cup coconut sugar
- 1 teaspoon molasses
- 2 Tablespoons paprika
- 2 Tablespoons Himalayan pink salt
- 1½ Tablespoons black pepper
- 1 teaspoon onion powder
- 1 teaspoon garlic powder
- 1 teaspoon celery powder
- ½ teaspoon cayenne powder

DIRECTIONS

1. Combine all ingredients in a mason jar.
2. Use a generous amount to rub on pork before baking, slow cooking or smoking.

GREEK TZATZIKI SAUCE

INGREDIENTS

- 1½ cups plain Greek yogurt
- 2 Tablespoons olive oil
- 1 medium cucumber, shredded with a box grater (about 2 cups)
- 1 Tablespoon fresh mint
- 1 Tablespoon lemon juice
- 1 teaspoon minced garlic
- ½ teaspoon salt

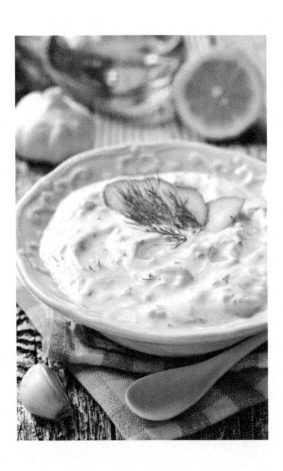

DIRECTIONS

1. Shred the cucumber using a box grater with large holes, then sit it in a colander for a few minutes to allow the juices to drain.
2. In a bowl, combine the Greek yogurt, olive oil, mint, lemon juice, garlic, and salt and mix together.
3. Add the shredded cucumber and mix again.
4. Serve or store in the fridge for later.

NOTES

Tzatziki is great as a dip with fresh vegetables, grilled kabobs, or chicken or as a saucy addition to a salad or protein bowl. Tzatziki keeps well in the fridge for about 4 days.

NUTRITION (FOR 2 TABLESPOONS)

Calories: 20 | Total Fat: 1 g | Total Carbs: 1 g
Protein: 1 g

COOK TIME: 0 MIN
PREP TIME: 5 MIN
SERVINGS: 4

CHICKPEA HUMMUS

INGREDIENTS

- 1 (15-ounce) can of chickpeas or garbanzo beans (no salt added)
- 3 Tablespoons lemon juice
- 2 Tablespoons tahini
- 2 garlic cloves or 2 teaspoons minced garlic
- ½ teaspoon salt
- 1 Tablespoon olive oil
- ¼ - ½ teaspoon paprika for serving
- Olive oil for serving
- Fresh parsley for serving

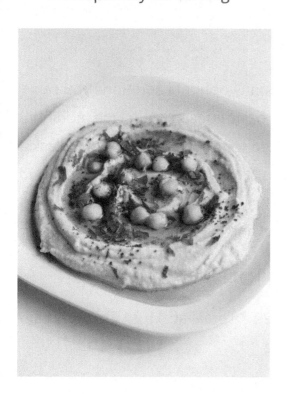

DIRECTIONS

1. Dump the canned chickpeas into a bowl and cover with water. Rub the chickpeas with your fingers to peel the skin off, then strain them in a colander and add them to a food processor.
2. Blend the chickpeas in the food processor until smooth.
3. Add the lemon juice, tahini, garlic, salt, and olive oil.
4. Blend in the food processor until smooth and creamy. Adjust the taste to your liking by adding more lemon juice, salt, and garlic if desired.
5. To serve, add the hummus to a bowl and drizzle on olive oil, sprinkle with paprika, and garnish with fresh parsley.
6. Store in the fridge for up to 1 week.

NUTRITION (FOR 2 TABLESPOONS)

Calories: 53 | Total Fat: 2 g | Total Carbs: 7 g
Protein: 2 g

COOK TIME: 0 MIN
PREP TIME: 5 MIN
SERVINGS: 4

GUACAMOLE

INGREDIENTS

- 2 large avocados
- 2 Tablespoons red onion, finely chopped
- 2 Tablespoons fresh cilantro, chopped
- 1 Tablespoon lime juice
- ¼ teaspoon salt

COOK TIME: 0 MIN
PREP TIME: 5 MIN
SERVINGS: 4

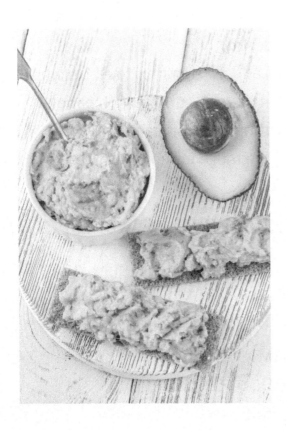

DIRECTIONS

1. Cut the avocados in half and remove the pits.
2. Use a knife to cut the avocado into cubes while it's still in the peel, then use a spoon to scoop out the avocado and add to a bowl.
3. Add the red onion, fresh cilantro, lime juice, and salt to the bowl and mix together. Use a fork to mash to desired consistency.
4. Add more red onion, cilantro, lime juice, and/or salt to desired taste.
5. Serve immediately or store in the fridge.

NOTES

There are many optional additions you can add to this basic guacamole recipe. Additions include diced tomato, diced jalapeño, black beans, corn, fresh basil, pineapple, sun-dried tomatoes, Kalamata olives, bacon, crumbled feta cheese, and salsa.

NUTRITION

Calories: 122 | Total Fat: 11 g | Total Carbs: 7 g
Protein: 2 g

CHAPTER 3
BREAKFAST

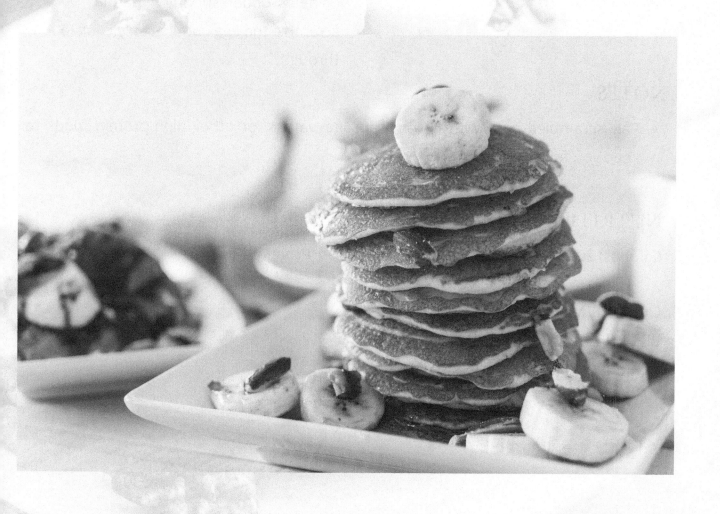

SIMPLE SCRAMBLED EGGS

INGREDIENTS

- 1 Tablespoon olive or avocado oil
- 4 eggs

Optional additions:
- Feta cheese
- Nutritional yeast
- Diced veggies
- Diced ham
- Crumbled bacon

DIRECTIONS

1. Set your stovetop burner to low-medium heat.
2. Whisk up the 2 eggs in a measuring cup.
3. Add in any high-fat, high-protein, low-carb options you choose.
4. Add the olive or avocado oil to the skillet and allow it to disperse evenly over the pan.
5. Pour in the scrambled egg mixture and, using a wooden spoon or spatula, scramble the eggs until evenly cooked through.

NOTES

- Pair scrambled eggs with bacon, sausage patties, or other high-protein foods to keep you full all morning.

NUTRITION

Calories: 203 | Total Fat: 16 g | Total Carb: 1 g | Protein: 13 g

COOK TIME: 5 MIN
PREP TIME: 5 MIN
SERVINGS: 2

MEDITERRANEAN SCRAMBLED EGGS

INGREDIENTS

- 4 eggs
- 1 Tablespoon olive or avocado oil
- 4 Tablespoons crumbled feta
- 4 Tablespoons diced tomatoes
- Fresh parsley to garnish
- Optional additions: black or green olives, chopped green onion, sun-dried tomato, diced bell peppers, black beans, etc.

COOK TIME: 5 MIN
PREP TIME: 5 MIN
SERVINGS: 2

NUTRITION

Calories: 244 | Total Fat: 19 g | Total Carb: 2 g | Protein: 15 g

DIRECTIONS

1. Set your stovetop burner to low-medium heat.
2. Whisk up the 2 eggs in a measuring cup.
3. Add the crumbled feta, diced tomatoes, fresh parsley, and any other additions you have to the scrambled egg mixture.
4. Add the olive or avocado oil to the skillet and allow it to spread evenly over the pan.
5. Pour in the scrambled egg mixture and, using a wooden spoon or spatula, scramble the eggs until evenly cooked through.

CLASSIC BREAKFAST FRITTATA

INGREDIENTS

- 1 Tablespoon olive oil
- 4 eggs
- 4 pieces cooked bacon or ham (nitrate free)
- ½ cup finely diced vegetables of choice (onions and mushrooms are great options)
- ¼ cup crumbled feta cheese
- Fresh herbs, chopped (parsley and basil are great choices)

COOK TIME: 10 MIN
PREP TIME: 5 MIN
SERVINGS: 2

DIRECTIONS

1. Set your stovetop burner to low-medium heat.
2. Whisk up the 4 eggs in a measuring cup.
3. Coat the frying pan with the olive oil, then pour the scrambled eggs onto the frying pan.
4. Sprinkle the diced vegetables and cheese on top, then place the cover over the frying pan.
5. Let the frittata cook with the lid on for 5-10 minutes until the top of the frittata looks formed and there is no liquid egg.
6. Remove the lid, then sprinkle on the fresh herbs.
7. Allow to sit for a minute, then serve.

NOTES

- Double or triple the recipe and use a larger skillet to make more servings. This frittata freezes well and can be reheated quickly in the microwave for a delicious, high-protein breakfast.

NUTRITION

Calories: 353 | Total Fat: 27 g | Total Carb: 3 g | Protein: 24 g
*Calories vary depending on the meat, vegetables, and cheese used.

GREEK VEGETABLE & FETA FRITTATA

INGREDIENTS

- 1 Tablespoon olive oil
- 4 eggs
- ½ cup spinach
- 6 cherry tomatoes, cut in half
- ¼ cup onion, finely chopped
- ¼ cup mushrooms, finely chopped
- 2 teaspoons fresh crushed garlic
- 6 green olives
- ¼ cup feta cheese
- Fresh or dried basil

COOK TIME: 10 MIN
PREP TIME: 5 MIN
SERVINGS: 2

NUTRITION

Calories: 297 | Total Fat: 21 g | Total Carb: 10 g | Protein: 5 g

DIRECTIONS

1. Set the stovetop burner to low-medium heat.
2. In a measuring cup, whisk together the eggs.
3. Coat the skillet with the olive oil, then add the scrambled eggs to the skillet.
4. Set the vegetables and feta cheese on top of the eggs, then place a lid on top of the skillet.
5. Let the frittata cook with the lid on for 5-10 minutes, until the top of the frittata is formed and there is no liquid egg.
6. Remove the lid and add the fresh or dried basil.
7. Serve immediately or store in the fridge or freezer.

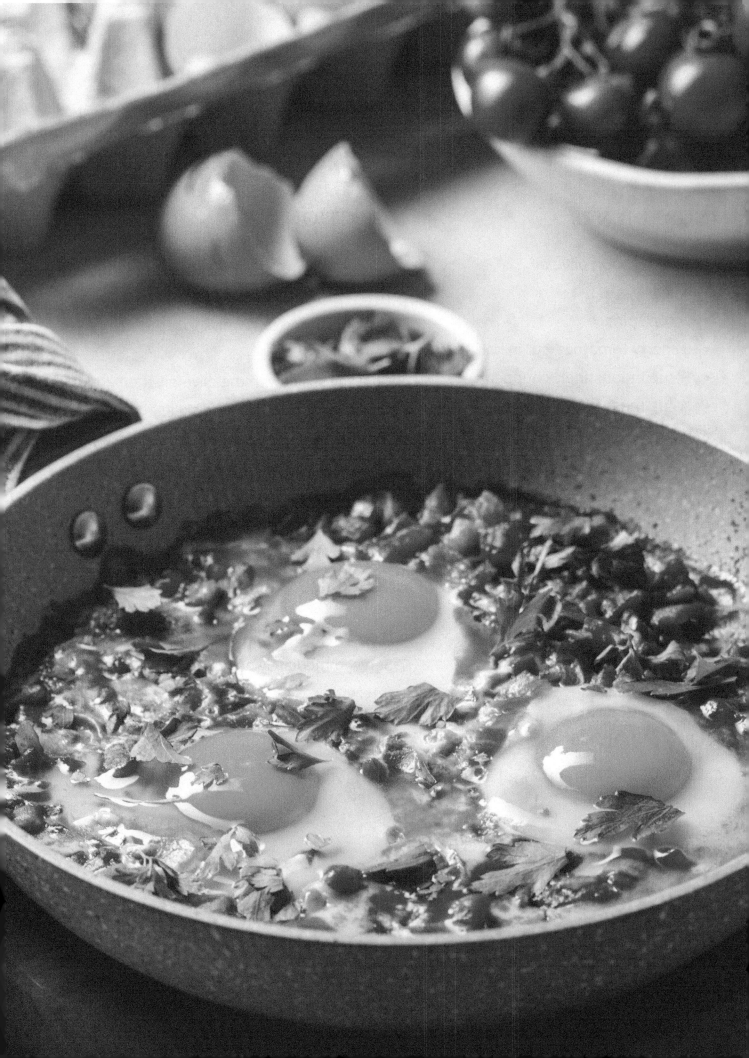

WHITE BEANS & EGGS IN PURGATORY

INGREDIENTS

- 2 Tablespoons olive oil or avocado oil
- 1 small yellow onion, chopped
- 2 cloves garlic, minced (about 2 teaspoons)
- 1 (28-ounce) can of whole peeled tomatoes
- 1-2 teaspoons red pepper flakes
- ½ teaspoon oregano
- ½ teaspoon paprika
- salt and pepper
- 1 (15-ounce) can cannellini beans, drained and rinsed
- 6 eggs
- 2 Tablespoons fresh parsley, chopped

COOK TIME: 25 MIN
PREP TIME: 5 MIN
SERVINGS: 3

NUTRITION

Calories: 487 | Total Fat: 19 g | Total Carb: 37 g | Protein: 24 g

DIRECTIONS

1. In a large pan, add the olive oil, onion, and garlic. Cook over medium heat until the onion becomes soft.
2. Add the red pepper flakes, oregano, paprika, salt, and pepper, and reduce the heat to a low setting.
3. Using a food processor, puree the whole peeled tomatoes until they look finely "chopped."
4. Add the tomatoes to the pot and mix, allowing them to simmer.
5. Add the cannellini beans and allow to simmer for 10-15 minutes.
6. Make 6 small wells in the sauce, then crack the eggs into each of the wells.
7. Set the stove to medium heat and allow to simmer until the whites of the eggs cook through.
8. Remove from heat, then garnish with fresh parsley.

SWEET POTATO & EGG SKILLET

INGREDIENTS

- 1½ Tablespoons ghee
- 1 large sweet potato, washed and cubed (about 2 cups)
- ½ red onion, diced
- 1 clove of garlic
- 2 cups spinach
- 4 eggs
- 1 teaspoon dried rosemary
- Salt & pepper to taste

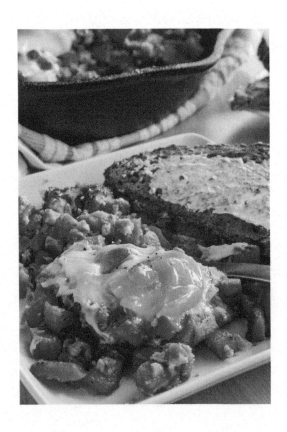

DIRECTIONS

1. In a skillet, add the ghee, diced sweet potatoes, red onion, and garlic cloves. Cook over medium heat until the vegetables are soft.
2. Add the spinach and mix thoroughly, allowing the spinach to become soft.
3. Crack the eggs and add to the top of the vegetables.
4. If you want your yolk to cook through, cover the skillet with a lid and allow it to cook for about 5 minutes. If you want your yolks to be "runny," do not cover them with a lid.
5. Season with rosemary, salt, and pepper, and serve immediately.

COOK TIME: 10 MIN
PREP TIME: 5 MIN
SERVINGS: 2

NUTRITION

Calories: 425 | Total Fat: 21 g | Total Carb: 45 g
Protein: 16 g

TRADITIONAL SHAKSHUKA

INGREDIENTS

- 3 Tablespoons olive oil or ghee
- 1 yellow onion, diced
- 1 red bell pepper, diced
- 1 cup mushrooms, diced
- 2 teaspoons minced garlic (about 4 cloves)
- 2 (14.5-ounce) cans diced tomatoes, one can drained of liquid
- 2 teaspoons paprika
- 1 teaspoon cumin
- ½ teaspoon chili powder
- ¼ teaspoon salt
- ¼ teaspoon pepper
- 6 eggs
- 1 bunch of fresh cilantro, chopped (about ½ - ¾ cup)

COOK TIME: 15 MIN
PREP TIME: 5 MIN
SERVINGS: 6

NUTRITION

Calories: 184 | Total Fat: 12 g | Total Carb: 11 g | Protein: 9 g

DIRECTIONS

1. Add the olive oil or ghee to a frying pan with the diced onion, bell pepper, mushrooms and garlic. Cook on medium heat until the vegetables are soft.
2. Add the diced tomatoes (with the juice of one can) to the pan and combine.
3. Add the paprika, cumin, chili powder, salt and pepper, then allow the dish to come to a simmer.
4. Using a spoon, make 6 small wells in the dish and crack an egg into each well.
5. Cover the pan with a lid and allow to cook for 6-8 minutes. If you want the yolks to be runny, remove the lid after 6 minutes. If you want the yolks to be more formed, allow the eggs to cook for closer to 8 minutes.
6. Top with the fresh cilantro (and feta cheese if your diet allows), then serve.

MEDITERRANEAN BREAKFAST BOWL

INGREDIENTS

- 4 eggs, scrambled
- 1 cup baby spinach
- ½ cup cherry tomatoes, cut in half
- ½ cup cucumber, cut in quarters
- 4 teaspoons fresh garlic
- 4 Tablespoons black or green olives
- 4 Tablespoons hummus
- 4 Tablespoons feta cheese

COOK TIME: 10 MIN
PREP TIME: 5 MIN
SERVINGS: 2

NUTRITION

Calories: 323 | Total Fat: 21 g | Total Carb: 11 g | Protein: 22 g

DIRECTIONS

1. Whisk two eggs and scramble in olive oil over low-medium heat.
2. Combine all other ingredients in a bowl and add to the cooked scrambled eggs.

SAVORY PORK SAUSAGE PATTIES

INGREDIENTS

- 1 pound ground pork
- 1 teaspoon dried rosemary
- 1 teaspoon dried sage
- 1 teaspoon dried thyme
- 1 teaspoon dried garlic powder
- 1 teaspoon dried onion powder
- 1 teaspoon salt

COOK TIME: 10 MIN
PREP TIME: 5 MIN
SERVINGS: 4

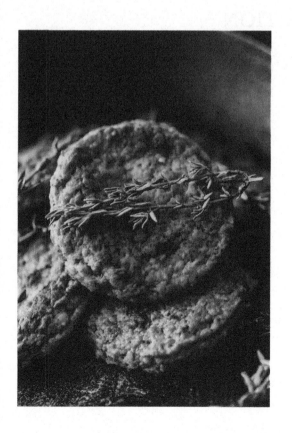

DIRECTIONS

1. Heat your skillet to low-medium heat.
2. In a mixing bowl, combine all ingredients and form 4 patties.
3. Coat your skillet with olive or avocado oil, then place the patties in the skillet.
4. Cook on each side for 2-4 minutes until completely cooked through.

NOTES

- These patties freeze well and are a great option for a quick and easy breakfast. Eat with two scrambled eggs and some roasted veggies, and you will be full all morning!
- When grocery shopping, look for pork that has at least 20% fat as you want some fat to help keep the patties from falling apart.

NUTRITION

Calories: 280 | Total Fat: 20 g | Total Carb: 0 g
Protein: 19 g

BASIC CHIA PUDDING

INGREDIENTS

- 1 cup unsweetened almond milk
- 6 Tablespoons chia seeds

COOK TIME: 30 MIN
PREP TIME: 5 MIN
SERVINGS: 2

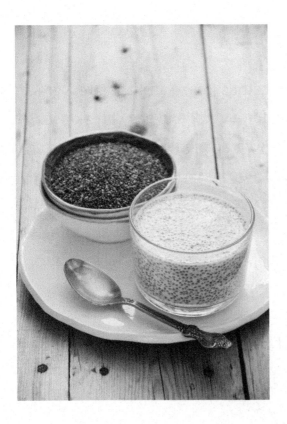

DIRECTIONS

1. In a small container or mixing jar, combine the almond milk and chia seeds.
2. Whisk together until the chia seeds are evenly distributed, then cover with a lid.
3. Place the chia pudding in the fridge and allow it to sit for at least 30 minutes. (Mixing halfway through encourages the chia seeds to stay evenly distributed.)
4. Top with your favorite healthy toppings and enjoy!

NUTRITION

Calories: 219 | Total Fat: 14 g | Total Carb: 18 g
Protein: 7 g

CHIA PUDDING COMBINATIONS

If you were to search for chia pudding recipes online, you would find endless varieties of toppings and tasty additions. Some additions are healthier than others, and I have listed my favorites here. Play around with the combinations and have fun, and be sure to write down some of your favorites to make again in the future.

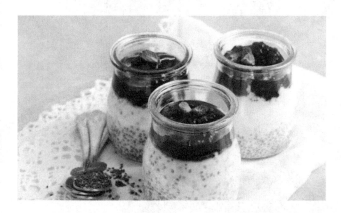

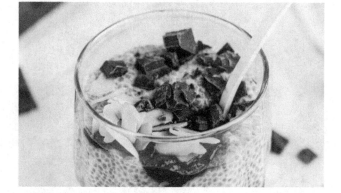

DELICIOUS ADDITIONS

- cocoa powder or shaved dark chocolate (look for over 75% cocoa)
- vanilla or almond extract
- cinnamon
- nutmeg
- almond butter, cashew butter, or peanut butter
- walnuts, pecans, sliced almonds
- berries: raspberries, blueberries, blackberries, strawberries
- coconut cream
- shredded unsweetened coconut
- honey or maple syrup

FAVORITE COMBOS

- cocoa powder and peanut butter
- cocoa powder, coconut cream, and shredded unsweetened coconut (tastes like an almond joy!)
- vanilla and cinnamon
- vanilla, raspberries, and chopped walnuts
- vanilla, strawberries, and pecans
- vanilla, coconut cream, and blueberries
- peanut butter and fresh blueberries or raspberries

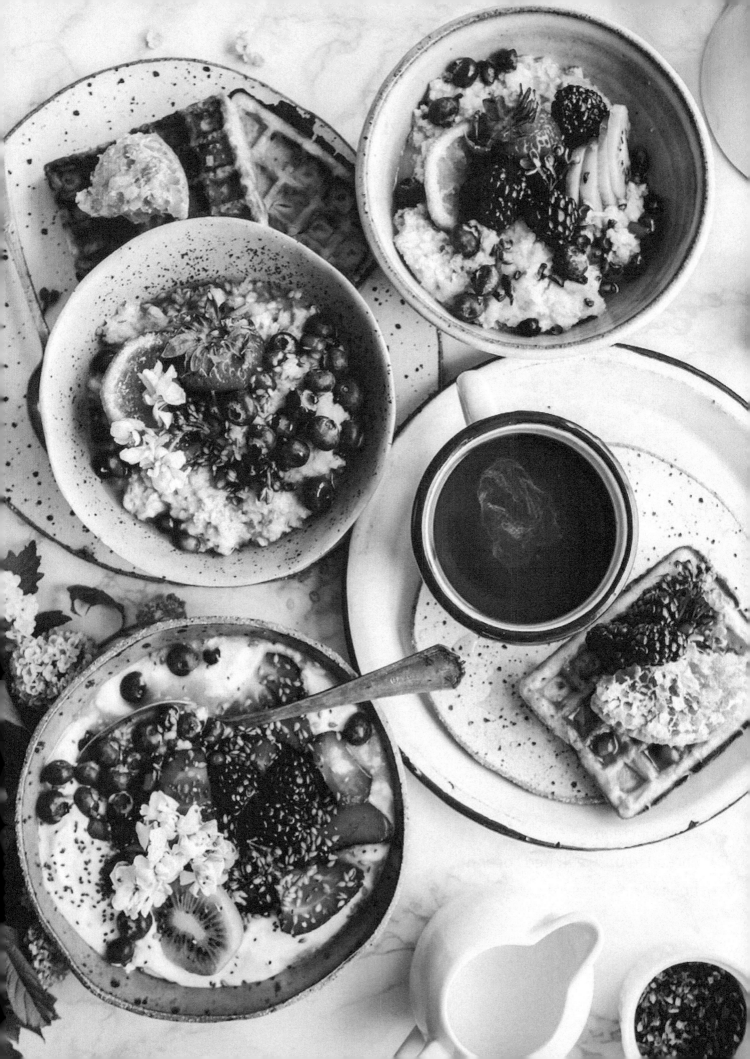

WAFFLES

A popular breakfast food in the United States, waffles can be a part of the Mediterranean diet when made with whole grains or nut-based flour and healthy toppings. The following basic waffle recipes are designed to match your personal preference and include whole grain, gluten-free, and low-carb options.

How to meal prep with waffles

The waffle recipes provided here are perfect for healthy meal prep as they freeze incredibly well. Allow them to cool completely before placing them in freezer bags and transferring them into the freezer. You can easily reheat each waffle by putting them in the toaster, making them nice and crisp for serving.

Fun and delicious toppings include:
- Fresh fruit including berries, apples, peaches, and pears
- Dried fruit including cranberries, raisins, and apricots
- Chopped pecans and walnuts
- Unsweetened coconut flakes
- Nut butter including almond, cashew, and peanut butter
- Semi-sweet chocolate chips
- Dippy or "sunny side up" eggs
- Local maple syrup or honey

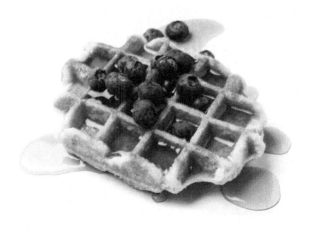

WHOLE WHEAT WAFFLES

INGREDIENTS

- 2 cups whole wheat flour
- 2 eggs
- 1¾ cup unsweetened almond milk
- ½ cup unsweetened applesauce (1 small applesauce cup)
- 4 teaspoons baking powder
- ¼ teaspoon salt
- 1 teaspoon real vanilla extract

COOK TIME: 10 MIN
PREP TIME: 5 MIN
SERVINGS: 8

NUTRITION

Calories: 150 | Total Fat: 3 g
Total Carb: 24 g | Protein: 6 g

DIRECTIONS

1. Turn on your waffle iron and allow it to warm up.
2. In a large mixing bowl, combine all of the ingredients and mix.
3. Spray the waffle iron, then using the ½ cup measuring cup, scoop the batter and pour it onto the waffle iron. You may need to use more or less than ½ cup of the batter for each waffle, depending on the size and shape of your waffle mold.
4. Allow the waffles to cook for 3-4 minutes, depending on the heat of your waffle iron. Check on your waffles after 3 minutes and adjust the time from there.
5. Transfer the cooked waffles onto a cooling rack or serve immediately.
6. For leftover waffles, allow them to cool on the cooling rack completely before transferring them to the fridge or freezer to prevent them from becoming soft and mushy.

GLUTEN FREE WAFFLES

INGREDIENTS

- 2 cups gluten-free flour
- 2 eggs
- 1¾ cup unsweetened almond milk
- ½ cup unsweetened applesauce (1 small applesauce cup)
- 4 teaspoons baking powder
- ¼ teaspoon salt
- 1 teaspoon real vanilla extract

COOK TIME: 10 MIN
PREP TIME: 5 MIN
SERVINGS: 8

NUTRITION

Calories: 160 | Total Fat: 2 g
Total Carb: 29 g | Protein: 4 g

DIRECTIONS

1. Turn on your waffle iron and allow it to warm up.
2. In a large mixing bowl, combine all of the ingredients and mix.
3. Spray the waffle iron, then using the ½ cup measuring cup, scoop the batter and pour it onto the waffle iron. You may need to use more or less than ½ cup of the batter for each waffle, depending on the size and shape of your waffle mold.
4. Allow the waffles to cook for 3-4 minutes, depending on the heat of your waffle iron. Check on your waffles after 3 minutes and adjust the time from there.
5. Transfer the cooked waffles onto a cooling rack or serve immediately.
6. For leftover waffles, allow them to cool on the cooling rack completely before transferring them to the fridge or freezer to prevent them from becoming soft and mushy.

LOW CARB WAFFLES

INGREDIENTS

- 2 cups blanched almond flour
- 2 eggs
- 1¾ cup unsweetened almond milk
- ½ cup unsweetened applesauce (1 small applesauce cup)
- 4 teaspoons baking powder
- ¼ teaspoon salt
- 1 teaspoon real vanilla extract

COOK TIME: 10 MIN
PREP TIME: 5 MIN
SERVINGS: 8

NUTRITION

Calories: 220 | Total Fat: 17 g
Total Carb: 8 g | Protein: 8 g

DIRECTIONS

1. Turn on your waffle iron and allow it to warm up.
2. In a large mixing bowl, combine all of the ingredients and mix.
3. Spray the waffle iron, then using the ½ cup measuring cup, scoop the batter and pour it onto the waffle iron. You may need to use more or less than ½ cup of the batter for each waffle, depending on the size and shape of your waffle mold.
4. Allow the waffles to cook for 3-4 minutes, depending on the heat of your waffle iron. Check on your waffles after 3 minutes and adjust the time from there.
5. Transfer the cooked waffles onto a cooling rack or serve immediately.
6. For leftover waffles, allow them to cool on the cooling rack completely before transferring them to the fridge or freezer to prevent them from becoming soft and mushy.

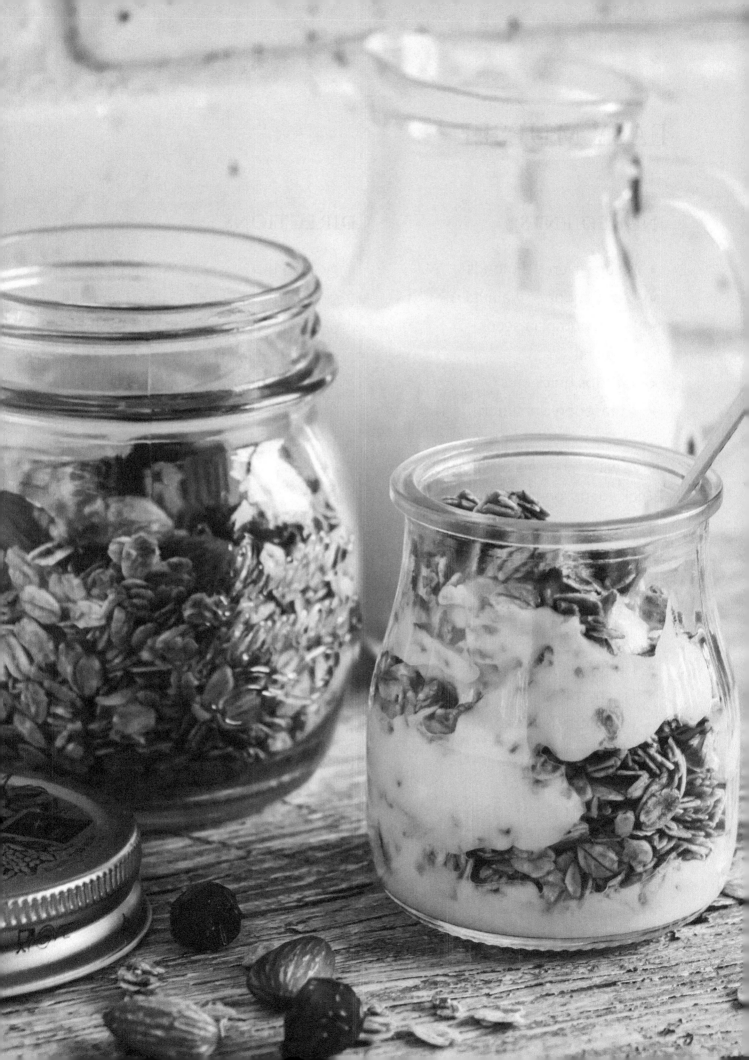

EASY MUESLI

INGREDIENTS

- ½ cup slivered almonds
- ½ cup chopped walnuts
- ⅓ cup pumpkin seeds (pepitas)
- 1½ cups quick oats
- 1 teaspoon cinnamon

Serve with ¾ cup plain, whole Greek yogurt per serving.

Other toppings include:
- Honey
- Maple syrup
- Unsweetened coconut flakes
- Dried fruit pieces
- Fresh fruit
- Nut butter (almond, peanut, cashew, etc.)

DIRECTIONS

1. Preheat the oven to 325 degrees F.
2. Spread the almonds, walnuts, and pumpkin seeds on a sheet pan and toast in the oven for 10 minutes.
3. Remove and allow to cool, then add the quick oats and cinnamon.
4. Transfer to an airtight container for storage.

For serving with ¾ cup Greek yogurt:

1. Top the Greek yogurt with ¼ cup muesli mix.
2. Add additional toppings of your choosing, such as fresh berries and local honey.

COOK TIME: 10 MIN
PREP TIME: 5 MIN
SERVINGS: 12

NUTRITION

Calories: 110 | Total Fat: 7 g | Total Carb: 9 g | Protein: 3 g

*Nutrition varies based on additional toppings added. The nutrition info provided is for ¼ cup muesli, not including Greek yogurt and additional toppings.

EASY BANANA PANCAKES

INGREDIENTS

- 2 bananas
- 2 whole eggs
- 2 egg whites
- 1-2 teaspoons vanilla (to taste)
- Cinnamon

Optional toppings:
- Maple syrup
- Honey (local is best)
- Peanut butter or other nut butter

COOK TIME: 5 MIN
PREP TIME: 5 MIN
SERVINGS: 2

NUTRITION

Calories: 185 | Total Fat: 5 g
Total Carb: 28 g | Protein: 10 g

DIRECTIONS

1. In a small bowl, mash the banana with a fork.
2. Add the whole eggs and egg whites and mix until thoroughly combined.
3. Add the vanilla and mix again.
4. Using a ⅓ cup measuring spoon, add the pancake mix to a skillet. Sprinkle cinnamon on top of each pancake.
5. Cook over medium heat until the center starts to form and doesn't look as runny.
6. Flip the pancakes and allow to cook for 3-4 minutes.
7. Remove from the skillet and serve with your favorite toppings for a filling breakfast.

NOTES

- You can easily double or triple this recipe to serve more people or freeze for later.
- Allow the pancakes to cool completely before transferring them to a freezer-safe container or bag and placing them in the freezer.
- To thaw, allow them to thaw in the fridge overnight or place them in the toaster for a quick and easy breakfast.

AVOCADO TOAST & EGGS

INGREDIENTS

- 2 slices whole grain or gluten-free bread, toasted
- 1 avocado
- 6 cherry tomatoes, cut in halves (optional)
- 4 eggs
- 1 Tablespoon olive oil
- Salt and pepper

COOK TIME: 5 MIN
PREP TIME: 5 MIN
SERVINGS: 2

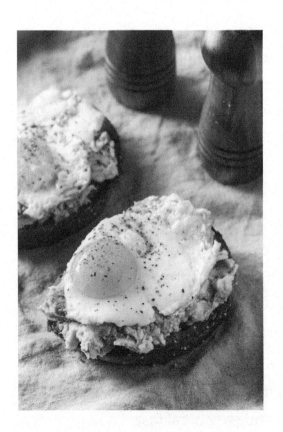

DIRECTIONS

1. Toast a piece of whole grain or gluten-free bread.
2. Cut an avocado in half and remove the pit.
3. Using a knife, cut the avocado into chunks while still in the peel.
4. Use a spoon to scoop out the avocado and add it to a bowl. Use a fork to slightly mash up the avocado, then spread the mashed avocado onto the toasted bread.
5. Add the halved cherry tomatoes to the avocado and toast.
6. In a small skillet, add the olive oil and cook your eggs. Options include scrambling the eggs or keeping the yolks runny.
7. Once cooked, place the eggs on top of the avocado toast.
8. Season with salt and pepper and enjoy!

NUTRITION

Calories: 415 | Total Fat: 30 g | Total Carb: 23 g
Protein: 16 g

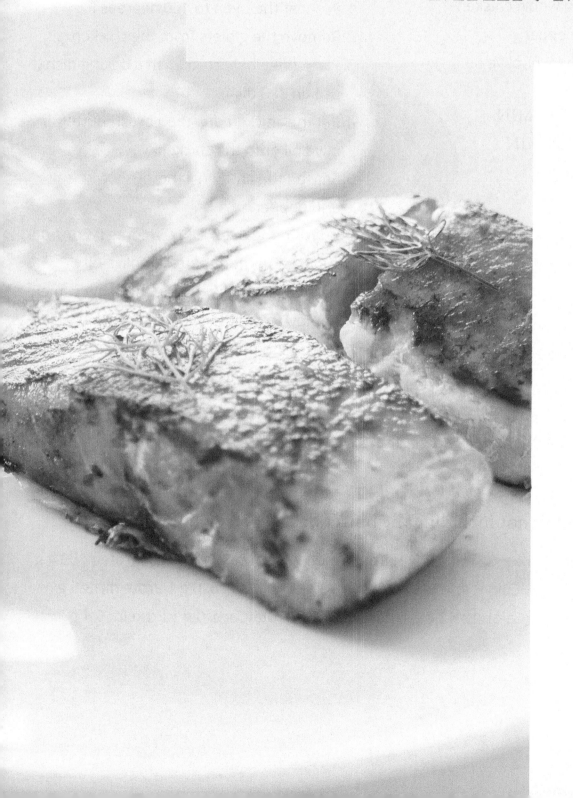

CHAPTER 4
MAIN MEALS

HOW TO ROAST A CHICKEN

INGREDIENTS

- 4-5 pound whole chicken
- Salt and pepper
- Butter, ghee, or olive oil

COOK TIME: 60 MIN
PREP TIME: 10 MIN
SERVINGS: 6+

NOTES

- A chicken is fully cooked when the thickest part reaches 165 degrees F.
- A general rule of thumb is to cook each pound of chicken for 15 minutes. So, if you have a 4-pound chicken, 4 x 15 = 60 minutes of cooking time.

DIRECTIONS

1. Preheat the oven to 400 degrees F.
2. Remove the giblets from the chicken.
3. Place the whole chicken in a baking dish (I use an 8x8 dish).
4. Pat the chicken dry, then brush butter or olive oil onto the chicken.
5. Season the chicken generously with salt and pepper.
6. Roast in the oven for 60 minutes. Consider rubbing on more butter or olive oil halfway through to make the skin crispier.
7. Remove from the oven and check the internal temperature to make sure it has fully cooked through (it should reach 165 degrees F).
8. Let the chicken rest for 15 minutes before serving.

NUTRITION (not including the butter or olive oil as amounts vary)

Chicken Breast, 3.5 oz: Calories: 284 | Total Fat: 6.2 g | Total Carb: 0 g | Protein: 53.4 g

One Chicken Thigh: Calories: 109 | Total Fat: 5.7 g | Total Carb: 0 g | Protein: 13.5 g

One Chicken Wing: Calories: 42.6 | Total Fat: 1.7 g | TotalCarb: 0 g | Protein: 6.4 g

COOKING CHICKEN FOUR WAYS

OVEN ROASTED

- Preheat the oven to 400 degrees F.
- Place the chicken (breasts or thighs) on a baking dish or sheet pan.
- Brush with olive oil and salt & pepper.
- Bake the chicken for 20-25 minutes, allowing the chicken to reach an internal temperature of 165 degrees F.

SLOW COOKER

- Pour about ¼ cup of chicken broth into the slow cooker, then add four pieces of chicken, laying in a single layer as best you can.
- Cook on low for 6-8 hours or high for 3-4 hours until the chicken reaches an internal temperature of 165 degrees F.

INSTANT POT

- Pour ½ cup water into the base of the instant pot, then place a trivet into the pot.
- Layer chicken (thighs or breast) into a single layer if possible.
- For every 1 pound of chicken, cook for 8 minutes in the instant pot using the "pressure cook" setting.
- Allow the Instant Pot to complete a slow release, or you can do a quick release if needed.

GRILLED

- Place chicken (thighs or breast) on the grill and season with olive oil, salt, and pepper.
- Cook on each side for 8-10 minutes or until the chicken reaches an internal temperature of 165 degrees F.

ITALIAN CHICKEN PATTIES

INGREDIENTS

- 1 pound ground chicken
- 1 egg
- 2 Tablespoons Italian seasoning
- 1 teaspoon garlic powder
- 1 teaspoon onion powder
- ¼ cup Parmesan cheese

COOK TIME: 10 MIN
PREP TIME: 5 MIN
SERVINGS: 4

DIRECTIONS

1. Heat the skillet to low-medium heat.
2. Combine all ingredients in a mixing bowl and divide into four equal-sized patties.
3. Coat the skillet with olive or avocado oil, then place the patties into the skillet.
4. Cook for 3-4 minutes on each side until evenly cooked through.

NOTES

- Top these chicken patties with marinara sauce and high-quality Mozzarella cheese.
- Add a side of roasted broccoli or green beans for a delicious, well-rounded meal.

NUTRITION

Calories: 226 | Total Fat: 14 g | Total Carb: 1 g | Protein: 24 g

BAKED MARGHERITA CHICKEN

INGREDIENTS

- 4 chicken breasts, boneless and skinless (about 1½ pounds total or 6 ounces for each breast)
- 2 Tablespoons olive oil
- 1 Tablespoon minced garlic
- 4 slices mozzarella cheese
- ½ cup basil pesto
- ½ cup cherry tomatoes, cut into halves
- ¼ cup fresh basil, chopped
- Salt & pepper to taste

COOK TIME: 20 MIN
PREP TIME: 5 MIN
SERVINGS: 4

NUTRITION

Calories: 577 | Total Fat: 42 g
Total Carb: 3 g | Protein: 47 g

DIRECTIONS

1. Preheat oven to 400 degrees F.
2. In a greased 8x8 baking dish, lay the chicken breast in a single layer.
3. Add the minced garlic and drizzle the olive oil on top of the chicken breasts, and use a brush to evenly coat the chicken.
4. Place a slice of mozzarella cheese over each chicken breast, then add roughly 2 Tablespoons of basil pesto on top of each breast.
5. Add the cherry tomatoes to the dish and add salt and pepper.
6. Bake in the oven for 20 minutes or until the chicken thighs reach an internal temperature of 165 degrees F.
7. Remove from the oven, garnish with fresh basil, and serve.

SPAGHETTI SQUASH CHICKEN MARINARA

INGREDIENTS

- 1 spaghetti squash
- Olive oil
- 4 chicken breasts, boneless and skinless (about 1½ lbs total or 6 ounces for each breast)
- 15 ounces marinara sauce (I recommend trying Rao's Homemade Marinara Sauce)

COOK TIME: 40 MIN
PREP TIME: 10 MIN
SERVINGS: 4

NUTRITION

Calories: 268
Total Fat: 11 g
Total Carb: 16 g
Protein: 26 g

DIRECTIONS

Bake the spaghetti squash

1. Preheat the oven to 400 degrees F.
2. Cut the spaghetti squash in half and scoop out the seeds with a spoon.
3. Drizzle with olive oil and lightly season with salt and pepper.
4. Place the squash face down on a lightly greased baking sheet and poke the skin a few times with a fork.
5. Roast for 40 minutes, then remove from the oven and flip the squash over to cool.
6. Use a fork to shred and pull up the strands of squash when ready to serve.

Cook the chicken

1. The chicken may either be roasted with the spaghetti squash or cooked in the skillet.
2. If baking, allow to cook for 20-25 minutes, then check to see if it is done. The internal temperature should be 165 degrees F.

Serve by creating a bed of spaghetti squash, then pour a small amount of marinara sauce over the squash and top with a chicken breast.

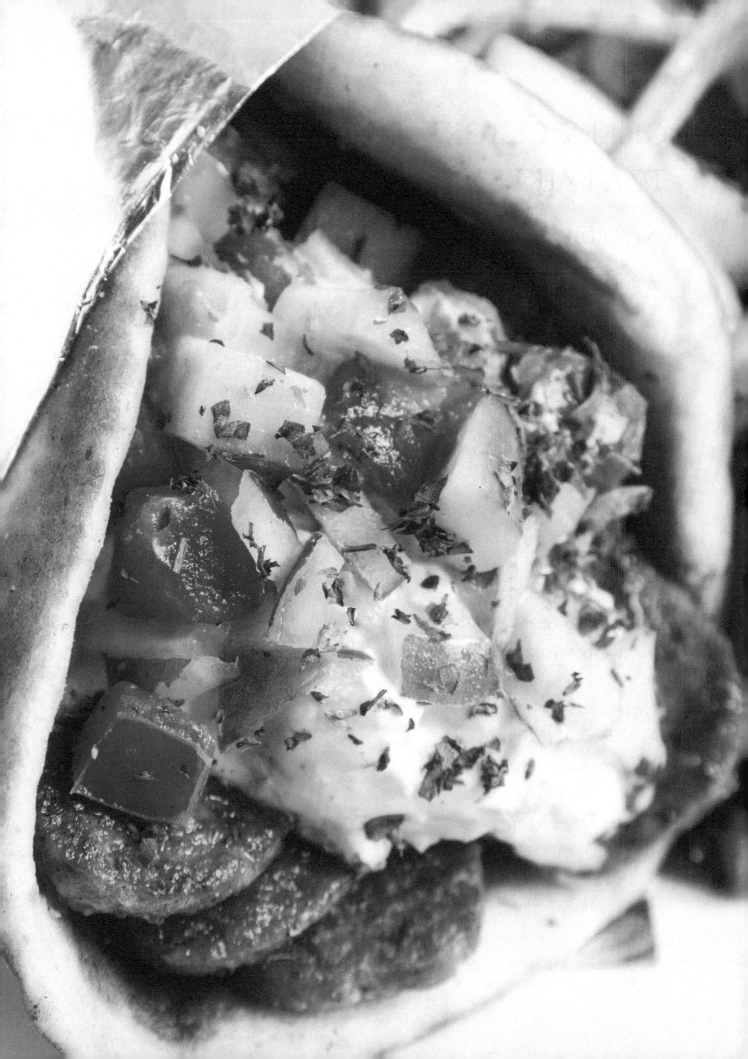

GREEK CHICKEN OR BEEF GYROS WITH TZATZIKI SAUCE

INGREDIENTS

Meat & Marinade

- 1 pound chicken breasts or beef, cut into strips
- 1 cup Greek yogurt (whole, plain)
- 2 Tablespoons olive oil
- 2 Tablespoons red wine vinegar
- 3 teaspoons minced garlic
- Salt and pepper to taste
- 1 Tablespoon oregano
- 1 teaspoon paprika
- 1 teaspoon cumin
- 1 teaspoon coriander

Gyro Fillings

- 4 pieces of pita bread
- Homemade Tzatziki Sauce (see recipe in Pantry Staples, Seasonings & Sauces section)
- 1 tomato, diced
- 1 cucumber, diced
- 1 red onion, cut into slivers
- Pitted kalamata olives
- Salt and pepper to taste

DIRECTIONS

- Combine all the marinade ingredients in a gallon ziplock bag and marinade in the fridge for at least 1 hour.
- Cook the chicken or beef strips in a skillet with olive oil over medium heat until fully cooked.
- Lay out your pita bread, then add tzatziki sauce, tomato, cucumber, red onion, olives, and your meat of choice. Season with salt and pepper, then fold the pita bread and serve.

COOK TIME: 15 MIN
PREP TIME: 1 HR 10 MIN
SERVINGS: 4

NUTRITION (USING CHICKEN)

Calories: 427 | Total Fat: 14 g
Total Carb: 40 g | Protein: 33 g

ITALIAN SAUSAGE WITH ZUCCHINI, FETA & QUINOA

INGREDIENTS

- 3 Tablespoons olive oil
- 12 ounces (4-5 links) Italian chicken sausage, cut into coins
- 2 small-medium zucchinis, about 2 cups chopped
- ½ cup crumbled feta cheese
- 1 cup dry quinoa
- 2 cups water
- Salt and pepper to taste
- Fresh basil to garnish

NOTES

For healthy chicken sausage links, I recommend Nature's Promise Mild Italian Chicken Sausage.

COOK TIME: 15 MIN
PREP TIME: 5 MIN
SERVINGS: 4

NUTRITION

Calories: 542 | Total Fat: 29 g | Total Carb: 37 g | Protein: 33 g

DIRECTIONS

1. Add the olive oil to a frying pan, then add the chicken sausage and zucchini and cook over medium heat. Cook until the zucchini becomes soft, but not mushy.
2. In a medium-sized pot, add the water and bring to a boil. Once the water is boiling, add the quinoa, allow the water to return to a bowl, then cover it with a lid. Turn the heat down to low and allow it to cook for about 10 minutes. Do not remove the lid at all during this time. Once you can see that the water has been absorbed by the quinoa, remove the lid and fluff it with a fork. Remove the pot from the stove.
3. Add the cooked quinoa to the skillet with the chicken and zucchini, then add the crumbled feta and allow it to melt into the dish.
4. Season with salt, pepper, and fresh basil and serve.

WHOLE ROASTED TURKEY

INGREDIENTS

- 10-pound turkey
- Salt and pepper
- Butter, ghee, or olive oil

COOK TIME: 60 MIN
PREP TIME: 10 MIN
SERVINGS: 6+

NOTES

- A turkey is fully cooked when the thickest part reaches 165-180 degrees F.

DIRECTIONS

1. Preheat the oven to 350 degrees F.
2. Remove the giblets from the turkey, rinse the inside and outside, then pat dry with a paper towel.
3. Use olive oil, ghee, or butter to brush the outside of the turkey.
4. Sprinkle with salt and pepper.
5. Roast for about 2 hours, then remove from the oven and allow to rest for at least 20 minutes. You may need to add additional time if the internal temperature is not yet 165 degrees F.

NUTRITION (does not include the olive oil, ghee, or butter)

Turkey Breast, 3 oz: Calories: 117 | Total Fat: 2 g | Total Carb: 0 g | Protein: 24 g

BAKED TURKEY, ZUCCHINI, SPINACH & FETA CASSEROLE

INGREDIENTS

- 2 Tablespoons olive oil (separated)
- 1 pound ground turkey
- 2 small yellow squash, diced
- 2 small zucchinis, diced
- 3 cups baby spinach
- ½ cup feta cheese
- Salt & pepper to taste

COOK TIME: 30 MIN
PREP TIME: 5 MIN
SERVINGS: 4

NUTRITION

Calories: 359 | Total Fat: 17 g
Total Carb: 18 g | Protein: 32 g

DIRECTIONS

1. Preheat the oven to 400 degrees F.
2. In a medium-sized saucepan, add 1 Tablespoon of olive oil and the ground turkey, Cook over medium heat until the meat is fully cooked and browned. Transfer the meat to a small bowl and set aside.
3. In the saucepan, add the diced yellow squash and zucchini with 1 Tablespoon olive oil. Cook over medium heat until the squash becomes soft, then add the baby spinach and allow it to wilt.
4. Add the ground turkey to the skillet to combine with the veggies, then transfer the mixture to a greased 8x8 baking dish.
5. Sprinkle feta cheese on top of the dish and season lightly with salt and pepper.
6. Bake for 15 minutes until the feta turns golden brown.
7. Remove from the oven and serve.

UNSTUFFED BELL PEPPERS

INGREDIENTS

- 1 pound ground turkey
- 1 green bell pepper, diced
- 1 red bell pepper, diced
- 1 red onion, diced
- 2 teaspoons Italian seasoning
- 3 cloves minced garlic
- 2 cups vegetable or chicken broth (low sodium)
- 1 (15-ounce) can of low-sodium diced tomatoes
- 1 (8-ounce) can of tomato sauce
- 1 cup quinoa, cooked
- Fresh parsley
- Avocado or guacamole

DIRECTIONS

1. In a large pot, combine the ground turkey, peppers, onion, Italian seasoning, and garlic. Cook until the meat is completely cooked through.
2. Add the broth, diced tomatoes, tomato sauce, and cooked quinoa, and bring to a simmer.
3. Serve with fresh parsley and avocado.

COOK TIME: 20 MIN
PREP TIME: 10 MIN
SERVINGS: 6+

HOW TO COOK QUINOA

- Bring 2 cups of water to a boil. Add 1 cup of quinoa to the boiling water, then allow it to return to a boil. Once the water is boiling, place a lid over the pot and turn down the temperature of the stove to low.
- Allow it to sit and cook for about 10 minutes or until all the liquid is absorbed. Do not remove the lid during this time as this will interfere with how the quinoa cooks.
- After about 10 minutes (once it looks like all of the liquid has been absorbed), remove the lid and fluff the quinoa with a fork.

NUTRITION

Calories: 247 | Total Fat: 8 g | Total Carb: 19 g | Protein: 23 g

MEDITERRANEAN PORK TENDERLOIN

INGREDIENTS

- 2 pounds pork tenderloin
- 2 Tablespoons olive oil
- 1 Tablespoon minced garlic
- ¼ cup balsamic vinegar
- 1 (8-ounce) jar of sun-dried tomatoes (I use Mezzetta's Julienne cut sun-ripened dried tomatoes)
- 4 ounces crumbled feta cheese
- Salt and pepper

COOK TIME: 25 MIN
PREP TIME: 5 MIN
SERVINGS: 8

NUTRITION

Calories: 303 | Total Fat: 14 g
Total Carb: 7 g | Protein: 36 g

DIRECTIONS

1. Preheat the oven to 400 degrees F.
2. Lightly grease a 9x13 baking dish.
3. Place the pork tenderloin in the baking dish, and cut the loin long ways down the middle.
4. In a small bowl, combine the olive oil, minced garlic, and balsamic vinegar, and lightly brush the mixture onto the pork loin.
5. Spoon the sun-dried tomatoes and crumbled feta cheese into the middle part of the pork loin that was cut.
6. Bake for 25 minutes or until the internal temperature of the pork is 145 degrees F.
7. Remove from the oven and allow to sit for 10-15 minutes before serving.
8. Season with salt & pepper to taste.

SLOW COOKER SPICED PULLED PORK

INGREDIENTS

- 4 pound pork butt or pork shoulder
- 2 Tablespoons minced garlic
- Juice from 1 orange (or ½ cup orange juice)
- 1 teaspoon onion powder
- 1 teaspoon garlic powder
- 1 teaspoon salt
- 1 teaspoon black pepper
- ¼ teaspoon chili powder
- 3 teaspoons dried oregano
- 1 teaspoon smoked paprika
- 2 teaspoons thyme

COOK TIME: 8 HOURS
PREP TIME: 5 MIN
SERVINGS: 6+

DIRECTIONS

1. Place the pork butt into the slow cooker.
2. In a bowl, add the minced garlic, orange juice, and all of the spices and mix well.
3. Add the spice mixture to the slow cooker, making sure to evenly coat the pork.
4. Cook on low for 8 hours or high for 4-5 hours. The pork will be more tender if you cook it on low for 8 hours.
5. Once fully cooked, remove the pork shoulder from the slow cooker and transfer it to a bowl.
6. Shred the pork using two forks, and add some additional liquid from the slow cooker as needed to shred the pork.

NOTES

- Serve this recipe with a side of roasted sweet potato, broccoli, or our Brussels sprout slaw recipe.

NUTRITION (for a 4 ounce serving of pork)

Calories: 339 | Total Fat: 24 g | Total Carb: 2 g | Protein: 27 g

LOW CARB PIZZA BOWLS

INGREDIENTS

- 1 pound ground sausage
- 8 ounces sliced mushrooms
- ½ onion, diced
- 12 slices pepperoni, cut into quarters
- 13 ounces of pizza sauce (I use Rao's Homemade Pizza Sauce)
- 2 teaspoons red pepper flakes
- 1 cup shredded mozzarella cheese

COOK TIME: 10 MIN
PREP TIME: 5 MIN
SERVINGS: 4

NUTRITION

Calories: 455 | Total Fat: 35 g | Total Carb: 9 g | Protein: 29 g

DIRECTIONS

1. Cook the ground sausage, mushrooms, and diced onion in a skillet on medium heat until the sausage is fully cooked and the veggies are soft.
2. Add the pepperoni, pizza sauce, and red pepper flakes.
3. Divide into four servings and top with mozzarella cheese if desired.

NOTES

This recipe is pretty versatile and can be easily adapted. Try adding diced peppers or black olives, using different types of meat, and substituting mozzarella with different types of cheeses for a variety of flavor profiles.

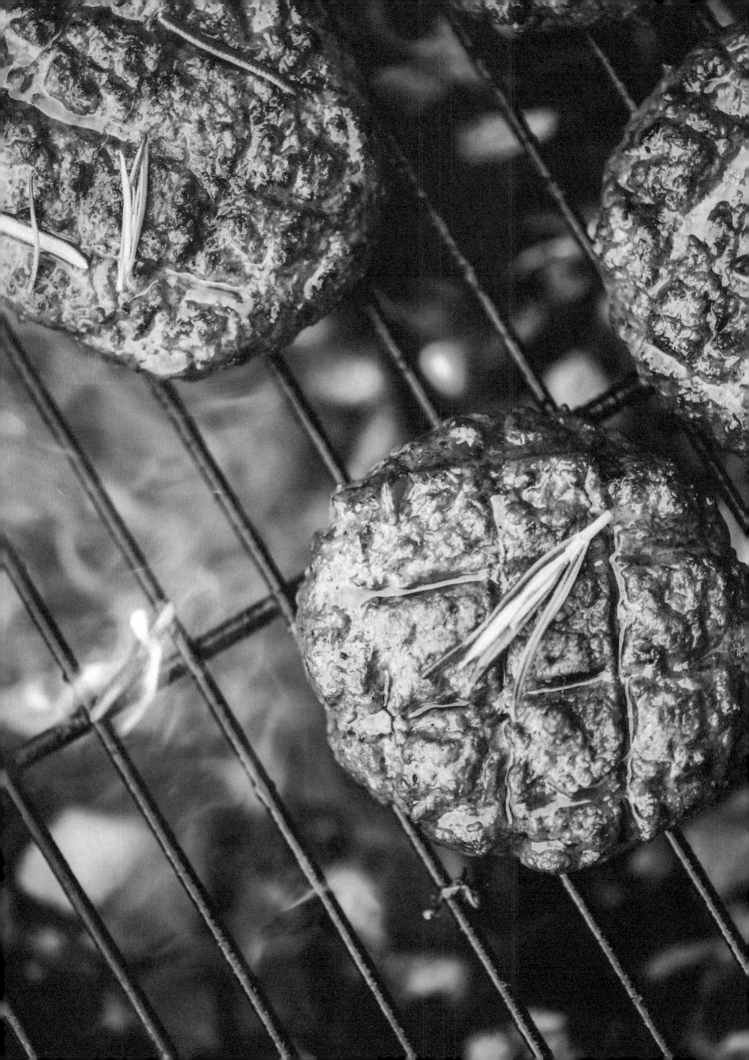

SIMPLE BEEF BURGERS

INGREDIENTS

- 1 pound ground beef (about 85% lean)
- 1 egg
- Salt & pepper
- 1 teaspoon onion powder
- 1 teaspoon garlic powder
- 1 clove fresh garlic, minced

COOK TIME: 15 MIN
PREP TIME: 5 MIN
SERVINGS: 4

NUTRITION

Calories: 218 | Total Fat: 13 g | Total Carb: 0 g | Protein: 25 g

DIRECTIONS

1. In a bowl, combine all ingredients and mix until well combined.
2. Divide the mixture into 4 even sized burgers.
3. Cook in a skillet or on the grill, about 5-7 minutes on each side, depending on how well done you prefer your burgers to be.
4. Serve on a bed of lettuce and diced tomatoes with ketchup or BBQ sauce.

STEAK & ONIONS

INGREDIENTS

- 1 pound beef or venison steaks
- 2 yellow onions, diced
- 4 Tablespoons butter, ghee, or olive oil
- Salt & pepper

COOK TIME: 10 MIN
PREP TIME: 5 MIN
SERVINGS: 4

NOTES

- Serve with a side salad to ensure you are enjoying plenty of vegetables.

NUTRITION

Calories: 238 | Total Fat: 15 g | Total Carb: 1 g | Protein: 26 g

DIRECTIONS

1. In a medium-sized skillet, add the butter, ghee, or olive oil.
2. Add the diced onions and saute until the onions are starting to get soft.
3. Sprinkle with salt and pepper.
4. Place the steaks on top of the onions and allow everything to cook together. Cook the steaks on each side for about 4-5 minutes.
5. Once the steak is cooked through and the onions are soft, remove them from the stove and serve.

GROUND BEEF STIR FRY

INGREDIENTS

- 1 pound ground beef (about 85% lean)
- 2 Tablespoons minced garlic
- 1 Tablespoon olive oil
- 1 bell pepper, diced (red, yellow, orange, or green)
- 1 cup cherry tomatoes, halved
- 2 cups baby spinach
- 1 teaspoon Italian seasoning
- ½ cup fresh shredded mozzarella
- Salt & pepper to taste

DIRECTIONS

1. In a skillet, add the ground beef, minced, garlic, and onion and cook over medium heat.
2. Once the meat is browned, add the diced bell pepper, cherry tomatoes, baby spinach, and Italian seasoning. Continue cooking until the veggies are soft.
3. Remove from heat, then add the mozzarella cheese and allow it to melt slightly before serving.
4. Season with salt and pepper as desired.

COOK TIME: 10 MIN
PREP TIME: 5 MIN
SERVINGS: 4

NUTRITION

Calories: 294 | Total Fat: 19 g | Total Carb: 4 g | Protein: 27 g

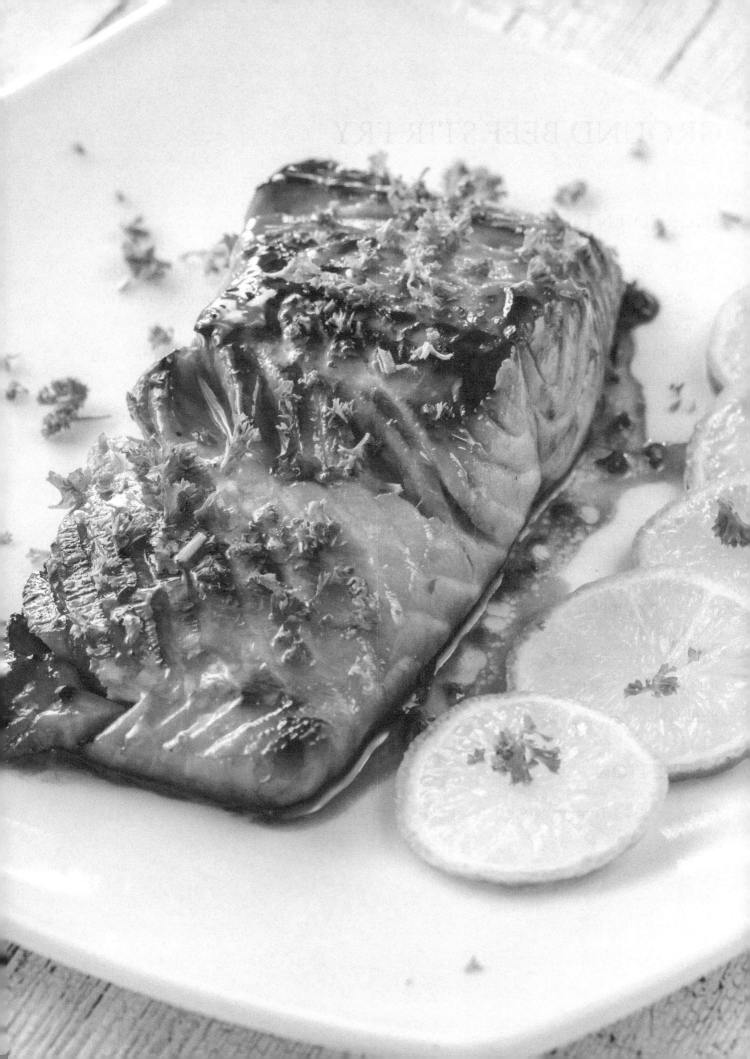

BAKED SALMON

INGREDIENTS

- 2-3 pound salmon fillet
- Olive oil for drizzling
- Salt & pepper

COOK TIME: 25 MIN
PREP TIME: 5 MIN
SERVINGS: 8-12

NUTRITION

Calories: 180
Total Fat: 9 g
Total Carb: 0 g
Protein: 23 g

DIRECTIONS

1. Preheat oven to 400 degrees F.
2. Place the salmon in a greased 9x13 baking dish.
3. Drizzle with olive oil and brush until evenly covered.
4. Season with salt and pepper.
5. Bake for 20-25 minutes, until the fish reaches an internal temperature of 145 degrees F.

SALMON & BROCCOLI WITH BALSAMIC REDUCTION

INGREDIENTS

- 2 cups balsamic vinegar
- ½ cup honey
- 2 pound salmon fillet
- 4 cups broccoli florets (fresh or frozen)
- Salt & pepper to taste

COOK TIME: 25 MIN
PREP TIME: 5 MIN
SERVINGS: 8

NUTRITION

Calories:391 | Total Fat: 16 g
Total Carb: 31 g | Protein: 29 g

NOTES

- Other vegetables to try in this recipe includes eggplant, zucchini, summer squash, onion, and cauliflower.

DIRECTIONS

1. Preheat oven to 400 degrees F.
2. In a medium-sized pot, add the balsamic vinegar and honey. Heat over medium-high heat until the mixture comes to a soft boil. Boil for about 15 minutes, stirring consistently, until the mixture becomes thick and has a "syrup-like" consistency.
3. Place the salmon in a greased 9x13 baking dish.
4. Lay the broccoli florets around the salmon, then drizzle about half of the balsamic reduction over the salmon and vegetables.
5. Season with salt and pepper, then bake for 20-25 minutes or until the fish reaches an internal temperature of 145 degrees F.
6. Remove from the oven, drizzle with additional balsamic reduction over the dish if desired, and serve.

BAKED TROUT

INGREDIENTS

- 2-3 pound trout fillet
- Olive oil for drizzling
- Salt & pepper
- Italian seasoning
- ¼ cup lemon juice
- 1-2 garlic cloves, minced

COOK TIME: 25 MIN
PREP TIME: 5 MIN
SERVINGS: 8-12

NUTRITION

Calories: 160
Total Fat: 7 g
Total Carb: 0 g
Protein: 23 g

DIRECTIONS

1. Preheat oven to 400 degrees F.
2. Place the trout fillet in a greased 9x13 baking dish.
3. Drizzle with olive oil and brush until evenly covered.
4. Season with salt, pepper, and Italian seasoning.
5. Bake for 20-25 minutes, until the fish reaches an internal temperature of 145 degrees F.
6. Combine the lemon juice and garlic cloves and lightly drizzle onto the fish for serving.

NOTES

- Other herbs that go well with trout include dill, parsley, sage, and chive.

TUNA CAKES

INGREDIENTS

- 8 ounces of canned tuna (in water), drained
- 2 eggs
- 2 Tablespoons olive oil-based mayonnaise (I use Primal Kitchen mayo)
- 1 Tablespoon Italian seasoning
- 2 garlic cloves, minced
- Salt & pepper to taste

NUTRITION

Calories: 123
Total Fat: 6 g
Total Carb: 1 g
Protein: 15 g

DIRECTIONS

1. Combine all ingredients in a bowl, then form into 4 patties.
2. Cook in a skillet with olive oil over medium heat, cooking for about 3 minutes on each side, then serve.

NOTES

- Serve these tuna patties on a bed of romaine lettuce with cherry tomatoes, celery, and cucumber with a balsamic vinegar dressing.

COOK TIME: 10 MIN
PREP TIME: 5 MIN
SERVINGS: 4

MEDITERRANEAN BAKED COD WITH ROASTED TOMATOES & ARTICHOKE

INGREDIENTS

- 1 pound of cod fillets (about 4 fillets)
- 1 Tablespoon olive oil
- 1 Tablespoon minced garlic
- 2 cups cherry tomatoes, halved
- 1 (15-ounce) can quartered artichoke hearts, drained
- ½ red onion, diced (about ½ cup)
- 4 ounces of kalamata olives
- ½ cup crumbled feta cheese
- Salt & pepper to taste
- Fresh basil, chopped (about ¼ cup)

COOK TIME: 25 MIN
PREP TIME: 5 MIN
SERVINGS: 4

NUTRITION

Calories: 292 | Total Fat: 18 g
Total Carb: 14 g | Protein: 19 g

DIRECTIONS

1. Preheat the oven to 375 degrees F.
2. In a greased 9x13 baking dish, lay the cod fillets in a single layer.
3. Combine the olive oil and minced garlic in a bowl, then use a brush to evenly apply on the cod.
4. Add the cherry tomatoes, quartered artichoke hearts, red onion, Kalamata olives, and crumbled feta cheese into the baking dish with the cod.
5. Lightly season with salt and pepper.
6. Bake for 20-25 minutes or until the cod flakes easily with a fork.
7. Remove from the oven, garnish with fresh basil, and serve.

NOTES

- This recipe is pretty versatile and can be made with a variety of vegetables. Try diced zucchini, summer squash, asparagus, broccoli, and cauliflower for different variations and flavors.

GREEK SHRIMP & FETA

INGREDIENTS

- 2 Tablespoons olive oil
- 1 yellow onion, diced
- 3 cloves garlic, minced
- 1 (28-ounce) can of diced tomatoes, drained
- 1½ teaspoons dried parsley
- 1½ teaspoons dried oregano
- ½ teaspoon red pepper flakes
- Salt & pepper to taste
- 1 pound of medium shrimp, fully cooked, deveined, tails removed
- 6 ounces of feta cheese, crumbled
- Fresh basil to garnish

COOK TIME: 25 MIN
PREP TIME: 5 MIN
SERVINGS: 4

DIRECTIONS

1. In a large skillet, add olive oil, diced yellow onion, and minced garlic and cook over medium heat. Allow the yellow onions to become soft.
2. Add the diced tomatoes, parsley, oregano, red pepper flakes, salt, and pepper.
3. Once simmering, add the shrimp and allow the shrimp to warm through.
4. Turn off the heat and add the feta cheese, allowing it to melt, then serve.

NOTES

- This dish goes great with quinoa or cauliflower rice.

NUTRITION

Calories: 316 | Total Fat: 14g
Total Carb: 10 g | Protein: 37 g

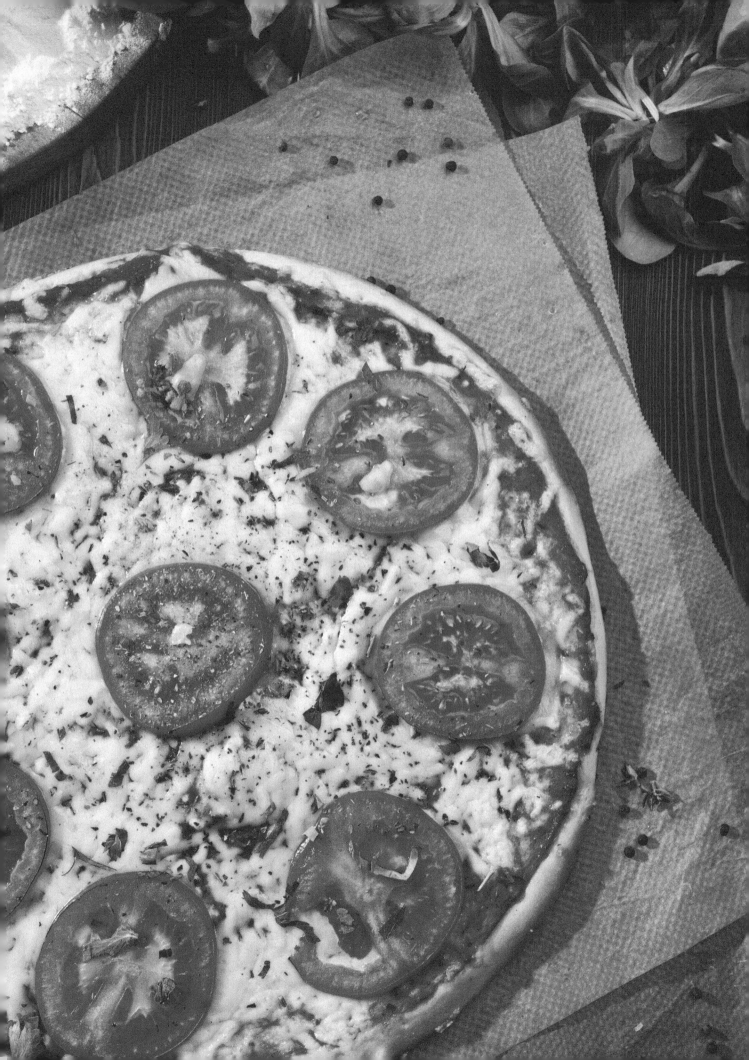

MARGARITA FLATBREAD

INGREDIENTS

- 1 naan bread or flatbread
- ¼ - ½ cup marinara sauce, depending on the size of the crust (I use Rao's Homemade Marinara Sauce)
- 1 cup fresh mozzarella
- 1 tomato, sliced very thin
- 3 garlic cloves, minced (about 1 Tablespoon)
- 2 Tablespoons olive oil
- 1 Tablespoon balsamic vinegar
- 6 fresh basil leaves

COOK TIME: 10 MIN
PREP TIME: 5 MIN
SERVINGS: 3

DIRECTIONS

1. Preheat the oven to 350 degrees F.
2. Lay the flatbread out on a greased baking sheet, then bake for 3-5 minutes to allow the flatbread to crisp up.
3. Remove from the oven, then top with marinara sauce, fresh mozzarella, and tomato.
4. In a small bowl, combine the minced garlic, olive oil, and balsamic, then drizzle over the flatbread.
5. Bake for about 10 minutes, until the crust is golden and the cheese is melting. Watch closely as the crust will brown up very quickly.
6. Remove from the oven and top with either whole or chopped basil.

NOTES

- For extra spice, add red pepper flakes.

NUTRITION

Calories: 367 | Total Fat: 23 g | Total Carb: 26 g | Protein: 13 g

MEDITERRANEAN FLATBREAD

INGREDIENTS

- 1 naan bread or flatbread
- ¼ - ½ cup marinara sauce, depending on the size of the crust (I use Rao's Homemade Marinara Sauce)
- ½ - 1 cup crumbled feta cheese
- 1 tomato, sliced very thin
- 3 garlic cloves, minced (about 1 Tablespoon)
- ¼ cup kalamata olives
- 1 handful of fresh spinach
- Fresh basil to garnish
- Optional: artichoke hearts, banana peppers

DIRECTIONS

1. Preheat the oven to 350 degrees F.
2. Lay the flatbread out on a greased baking sheet, then bake for 3-5 minutes to allow the flatbread to crisp up.
3. Remove from the oven, then top with marinara sauce, feta cheese, tomato, garlic, olives, and fresh spinach.
4. Bake for about 10 minutes, until the crust is golden and the cheese is melting. Watch closely as the crust will brown up very quickly.
5. Remove from the oven and top with either whole or chopped basil.

COOK TIME: 10 MIN
PREP TIME: 5 MIN
SERVINGS: 3

NUTRITION

Calories: 390 | Total Fat: 19 g | Total Carb: 32 g | Protein: 21 g

CARAMELIZED ONION & SPINACH FLATBREAD

INGREDIENTS

- 1 naan bread or flatbread
- ¼ - ½ cup marinara sauce, depending on the size of the crust (I use Rao's Homemade Marinara Sauce) OR Alfredo sauce (I use Primal Kitchen's Alfredo Sauce)
- 2 Tablespoons olive oil
- 1 cup red onion, sliced thinly
- 1 cup fresh spinach
- ½ - 1 cup crumbled feta cheese

COOK TIME: 10 MIN
PREP TIME: 5 MIN
SERVINGS: 3

DIRECTIONS

1. Preheat the oven to 350 degrees F.
2. Lay the flatbread out on a greased baking sheet, then bake for 3-5 minutes to allow the flatbread to crisp up.
3. In a small saucepan, combine the olive oil and red onion. Sauté for a few minutes until the onion becomes soft.
4. Remove the flatbread from the oven, then top with sauce, caramelized onion, spinach, and feta cheese.
5. Bake for about 10 minutes, until the crust is golden and the cheese is melting. Watch closely as the crust will brown up very quickly.
6. Remove from the oven and serve.

NUTRITION

Calories: 430 | Total Fat: 25 g | Total Carb: 28 g | Protein: 20 g

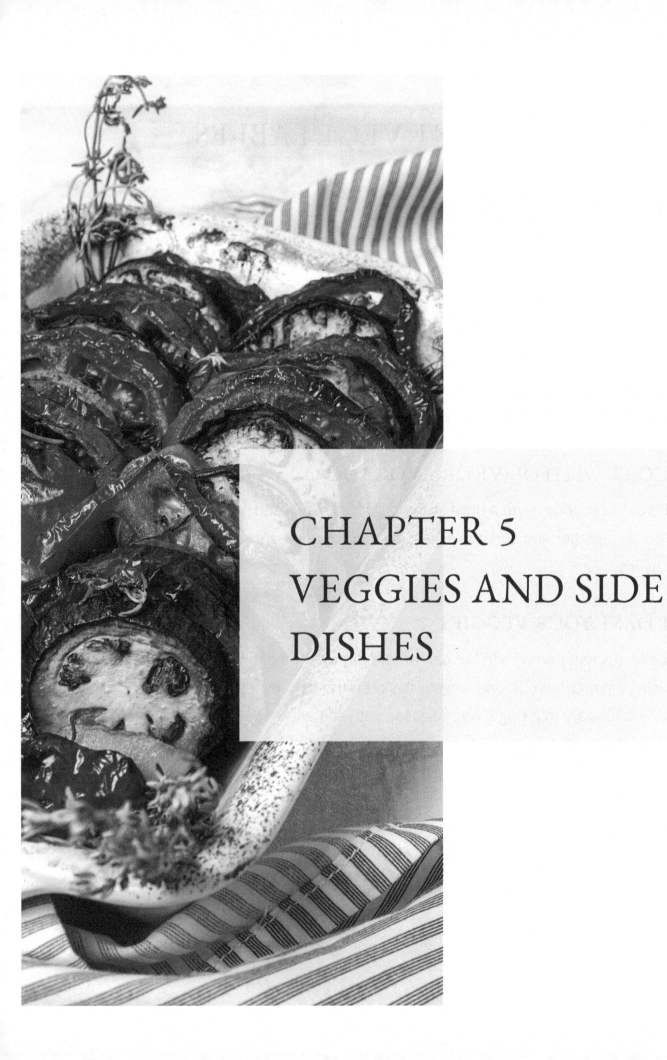

CHAPTER 5
VEGGIES AND SIDE DISHES

HOW TO ROAST VEGETABLES

CHOOSE YOUR VEGGIES

Choose any vegetable you would like or have on hand! The beauty of roasting vegetables is that you can mix and match, creating endless varieties!

SLICE, DICE, AND QUARTER

The most important thing to remember here is that every piece of vegetable should be about the same size. This will ensure the vegetables roast at the same rate and avoiding one vegetable from overcooking.

COAT WITH OLIVE OR AVOCADO OIL

Place the vegetables in a bowl and pour olive or avocado oil liberally over the veggies. Mix all together and add more oil as needed to make sure all the vegetables are covered.

ROAST YOUR VEGGIES

Cover a sheet pan with foil or parchment paper, then dab with olive or avocado oil using a paper towel. Dump vegetables onto the pan and spread them out so that the vegetables are in a single layer. Season with salt and pepper. Roast vegetables according to the next page's roasting time.

ROASTING TIMES FOR VEGETABLES

- Roasting times are based on the oven set at **425 degrees F**.
- Evenly coat the vegetables with olive oil or avocado oil before roasting.
- Mix the vegetables with a spatula halfway through the cooking time.
- If using a variety of vegetables, start with the shortest duration of time and check on your vegetables frequently, mixing them up halfway through and as needed for even roasting.
- Cut the vegetables to about the same size in order to ensure the vegetables roast evenly and at the same rate.

Vegatable	How to Prep	Roasting Time at 425 F (218 C)
Asparagus spears	whole, bottoms trimmed	10-12 minutes
Beets	whole, pierced with a fork, wrapped in foil	60 minutes
Beets	cubed	30 minutes
Bell peppers	cut into strips	15-20 minutes
Broccoli	separated into florets	20-25 minutes
Brussels sprouts	trimmed and halved	20-25 minutes

Vegatable	How to Prep	Roasting Time at 425 F (218 C)
Carrots	cut into coins	20 minutes
Cauliflower	separated into florets	20-25 minutes
Eggplant	cubed	20-30 minutes
Green beans	whole	12-15 minutes
Mushrooms	whole or sliced	20-25 minutes
Onion (red, yellow, white, etc.)	diced or cut into wedges	18-20 minutes
Potato	whole, pierced with a fork	40-45 minutes
Potato	cubed	30 minutes
Pumpkin	cubed	30 minutes
Squash, acorn	cut in half, seeds removed	45-50 minutes
Squash, butternut	cubed	40 minutes

Vegatable	How to Prep	Roasting Time at 425 F (218 C)
Squash, spaghetti	cut in half, seeds removed	30-45 minutes
Sweet potato	whole, pierced with a fork	40-45 minutes
Sweet potato	cubed	30-35 minutes
Tomatoes (plum, cherry, etc.)	whole, cut in half, or cubed	30-40 minutes.
Zucchini	cubed	30 minutes

Make roasted vegetables your go-to side dish!
Not only are roasted vegetables easy to prepare, but they also go with nearly every type of protein and are a great way to meal prep large amounts of vegetables.
Healthy protein + roasted veggies = the perfect meal!

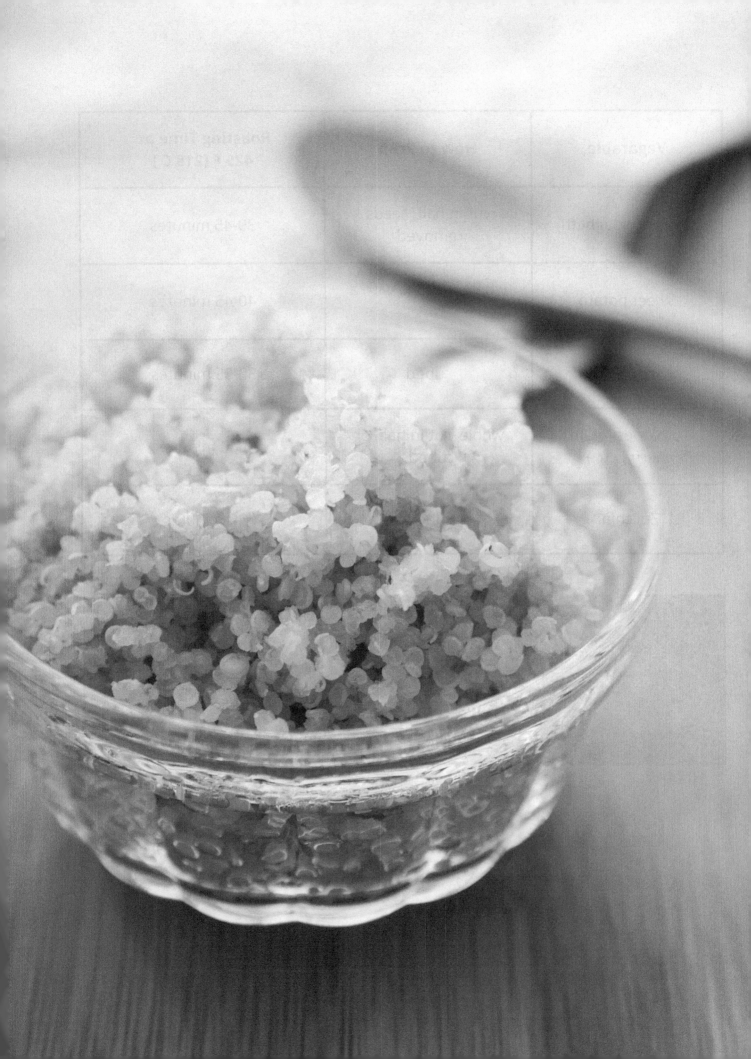

HOW TO COOK QUINOA

WHAT IS QUINOA?

Quinoa is a gluten free grain that is a complete protein, which means it contains all nine essential amino acids that our bodies are unable to make on its own. Quinoa is high in fiber, helps keep cholesterol and blood sugar levels in check, helps lower the risk of heart disease and diabetes, and is filled with antioxidants, B vitamins, and iron.

INGREDIENTS

- 2 cups of water
- 1 cup of quinoa

COOK TIME: 10 MIN
PREP TIME: 5 MIN
SERVINGS: VARIES

NUTRITION (for ½ cup cooked quinoa)

Calories: 110 | Total Fat: 2 g
Total Carb: 20 g | Protein: 4 g

DIRECTIONS

1. In a medium-sized pot, add the water and bring to a boil.
2. Once the water is boiling, add the quinoa, allow the water to return to a bowl, then cover the pot with a lid.
3. Turn the heat down to low and allow it to cook for about 10 minutes. Do not remove the lid at all during this time.
4. Once you can see that the water has been absorbed by the quinoa, remove the lid and fluff it with a fork.

NOTES

- The water-to-quinoa ratio when cooking quinoa is 2:1. So, 2 cups of water and 1 cup of dry quinoa makes 2 cups of cooked quinoa; 4 cups of water and 2 cups of dry quinoa make 4 cups of cooked quinoa, etc.
- This recipe's instructions can also be used to make delicious rice. Preparing rice also uses the 2:1 ratio.

ROASTED ZUCCHINI, ONION, TOMATO & FETA

INGREDIENTS

- 2 small zucchinis, cubed
- 1 pint cherry tomatoes, cut in halves
- 1 red onion, wedged or cubed
- 4 Tablespoons olive or avocado oil
- salt and pepper
- 3 ounces of feta cheese
- Fresh basil for garnish

COOK TIME: 10 MIN
PREP TIME: 10 MIN
SERVINGS: 3

NUTRITION

Calories: 298 | Total Fat: 24 g
Total Carb: 13 g | Protein: 7 g

DIRECTIONS

1. Preheat oven to 425 degrees F.
2. Prepare the vegetables, then mix them in a bowl with olive oil
3. Lay in a single layer on a sheet pan or a 9x13 baking dish.
4. Lightly season with salt and pepper, then sprinkle on the feta cheese.
5. Bake for 20-25 minutes until the vegetables are soft and the feta is slightly brown.
6. Garnish with fresh basil and serve.

NOTES

- This recipe is great on its own, or make it a complete meal by pairing it with roasted chicken and/or a serving of quinoa.

ROASTED EGGPLANT, ZUCCHINI, MUSHROOM & RED ONION BOWLS

INGREDIENTS

- 2 small zucchini, diced
- 1 small eggplant, diced
- 1 red onion, diced
- 1 pint sliced mushrooms
- 2 cups water
- 1 cup quinoa
- 4 ounces of feta cheese (about 1 cup)
- Fresh basil for garnish

COOK TIME: 10 MIN
PREP TIME: 10 MIN
SERVINGS: 4

NUTRITION

Calories: 373 | Total Fat: 29 g
Total Carb: 25 g | Protein: 11 g

DIRECTIONS

1. Preheat oven to 425 degrees F.
2. Prepare the vegetables, then mix in a bowl with olive oil and coat liberally.
3. Lay in a single layer on a sheet pan. (You may need to use two sheet pans.)
4. Lightly season with salt and pepper.
5. Bake for 20-25 minutes until the vegetables are soft.
6. In a medium-sized pot, add the water and bring to a boil. Once the water is boiling, add the quinoa, allow the water to return to a bowl, then cover it with a lid. Turn the heat down to low and allow it to cook for about 10 minutes. Do not remove the lid at all during this time. Once you can see that the water has been absorbed by the quinoa, remove the lid and fluff it with a fork. Remove the pot from the stove.
7. Serve the veggies with quinoa, feta cheese, and fresh basil.

BACON & BRUSSELS SPROUT SLAW

INGREDIENTS

- 4 cups Brussels sprouts, shaved using a food processor or knife
- 3 Tablespoons olive or avocado oil
- 8 strips cooked bacon, crumbled (nitrate free)
- ½ cup raw walnuts
- 2 Tablespoons fresh chive, chopped
- 3 Tablespoons lemon juice
- Salt and pepper to taste
- Red pepper flakes to taste

COOK TIME: 15 MIN
PREP TIME: 5 MIN
SERVINGS: 8

NUTRITION

Calories: 224 | Total Fat: 18 g | Total Carb: 9 g | Protein: 6 g

DIRECTIONS

1. Shred the Brussels sprouts using a food processor or knife.
2. Cook the bacon on the skillet or in the oven, allow it to cool, then crumble it into small pieces.
3. In a large, combine all ingredients and mix together.
4. Since warm or cold.

NOTES

- This dish is delicious served hot or cold. You may also add Parmesan or Mozzarella cheese.
- This dish is great on its own, or add additional protein such as ham or pork tenderloins.

LOADED MEDITERRANEAN POTATOES

INGREDIENTS

- 1 pound of red potatoes (about 8 potatoes), cut into bite-sized pieces
- ½ red onion, diced (about ½ cup)
- 2 Tablespoons olive oil
- 2 garlic cloves, minced (about 2 teaspoons)
- 1 Tablespoon dried rosemary or Italian seasoning
- 1 teaspoon thyme
- 1 teaspoon basil
- ½ teaspoon salt
- ½ teaspoon black pepper
- ½ cup crumbled feta cheese
- 8 ounces of chopped sun-dried tomatoes

DIRECTIONS

1. Preheat the oven to 425 degrees F.
2. In a bowl, add the red potatoes, red onion, olive oil, garlic, rosemary, thyme, basil, salt, and pepper. Mix until the potatoes are evenly coated with olive oil and spices.
3. Lay the potatoes out on a greased baking sheet. Add the sun-dried tomatoes and feta cheese to the sheet pan.
4. Bake for 20-30 minutes or until the potatoes are soft and golden brown.
5. Remove from the oven and serve.

COOK TIME: 20 MIN
PREP TIME: 5 MIN
SERVINGS: 6

NUTRITION

Calories: 204 | Total Fat: 9 g | Total Carb: 23 g | Protein: 5 g

RATATOUILLE

INGREDIENTS

- 1 medium eggplant, diced into cubes
- 1 zucchini, diced into cubes
- 1 yellow squash, diced into cubes
- 1 bell pepper (red, orange or yellow), cut into bite-sized pieces
- 1 red onion, chopped
- 3-4 Tablespoons olive oil
- 4 cloves garlic, minced (about 1 Tablespoon)
- 1 (14.5-ounce) can of diced tomatoes
- Handful of fresh basil, chopped
- 1 teaspoon red pepper flakes
- 1 teaspoon dried oregano
- Salt and pepper to taste

COOK TIME: 20 MIN
PREP TIME: 10 MIN
SERVINGS: 4

NUTRITION

Calories: 211 | Total Fat: 14 g
Total Carb: 19 g | Protein: 3 g

DIRECTIONS

1. Preheat the oven to 425 degrees F.
2. In a bowl, add the cubed eggplant and cover with a small amount of olive oil. Lay out on a greased baking sheet in a single layer.
3. Then, combine the zucchini, yellow squash, and bell pepper in a bowl. Add the olive oil and mix until the veggies are evenly coated with olive oil.
4. Lay out on a second greased baking sheet, making sure the veggies are spread out in a single layer. Season with salt and pepper.
5. Bake for about 15-20 minutes, until the veggies are soft and roasted.
6. While the veggies are roasting, add the chopped red onion and about 1 Tablespoon o olive oil to a pot.
7. Cook over medium heat on the stove until the onions become soft. Add the garlic and cook for 1 more minute.
8. Add the diced tomatoes to the pot and bring to a simmer.
9. Once the veggies are done roasting in the oven, add them to the pot on the stove. Allow to simmer for about 10 minutes, then add the fresh basil, red pepper flakes, oregano, salt, and pepper and mix together. Serve warm.

CHEESY SPINACH & MUSHROOM QUINOA

INGREDIENTS

- 2 cups water
- 1 cup quinoa
- 2 Tablespoons olive oil
- 2 (8-ounce) containers of sliced mushrooms (washed)
- 4 cups baby spinach
- 1 Tablespoon minced garlic
- 1 teaspoon red pepper flakes
- Salt and pepper to taste
- ¼ cup fresh basil, chopped
- ½ cup of your choice of cheese - feta, goat cheese, parmesan, or mozzarella are great choices

COOK TIME: 20 MIN
PREP TIME: 5 MIN
SERVINGS: 4

NUTRITION

Calories: 211 | Total Fat: 14 g
Total Carb: 19 g | Protein: 3 g

DIRECTIONS

1. In a medium-sized pot, add the water and bring to a boil. Once the water is boiling, add the quinoa, allow the water to return to a bowl, then cover the pot with a lid. Turn the heat down to low and allow it to cook for about 10 minutes. Do not remove the lid at all during this time. Once you can see that the water has been absorbed by the quinoa, remove the lid and fluff it with a fork. Remove the pot from the stove.
2. In a medium-sized pan, add the olive oil, sliced mushrooms. Cook over medium heat until the mushrooms become soft.
3. Add the baby spinach and allow it to wilt.
4. Add the garlic, red pepper flakes, salt, and pepper.
5. Remove the pan from the stove, then add the quinoa and mix well.
6. Garnish with fresh basil, add your choice of cheese to the top, and serve.

APPLE & PECAN STUFFED SWEET POTATOES

INGREDIENTS

- 4 medium sweet potatoes
- ¾ cup chopped pecans
- 4 Tablespoons butter or ghee
- 1 large red apple, diced
- ¼ cup golden raisins
- ½ teaspoon cinnamon
- ¼ teaspoon nutmeg

COOK TIME: 1 HR 20 MIN
PREP TIME: 5 MIN
SERVINGS: 4

NUTRITION

Calories: 437 | Total Fat: 31 g
Total Carb: 40 g | Protein: 4 g

DIRECTIONS

1. Preheat the oven to 425 degrees F.
2. Wash the sweet potatoes, then poke a few holes in each with a fork.
3. Place the sweet potatoes in the oven and bake for roughly 1 hour or until the potato feels tender when you insert a fork. You may need to add more time depending on the size of each potato. Once tender, remove the sweet potatoes from the oven and reduce the oven's temperature to 350 degrees F.
4. Add the chopped pecans to a small skillet and cook over medium-low heat, mixing them up continuously, for 2-3 minutes until toasted. Transfer the pecans to a small bowl and set aside.
5. Melt the butter in the skillet, then add the diced apples and raisins. Sauté until the apples are soft, then add the cinnamon and nutmeg. Remove from heat.
6. Once the sweet potatoes are done baking in the oven, cut them in half long ways, keeping the "shell" intact. Scoop out the insides with a spoon and transfer them to a bowl.
7. Add the apple mixture to the sweet potato pulp and thoroughly combine. Then, spoon the mixture back into the sweet potato shells.
8. Place the stuffed sweet potatoes on a baking sheet and bake at 350 degrees F for 15 minutes.
9. Remove from the oven, garnish with the toasted pecans, and serve.

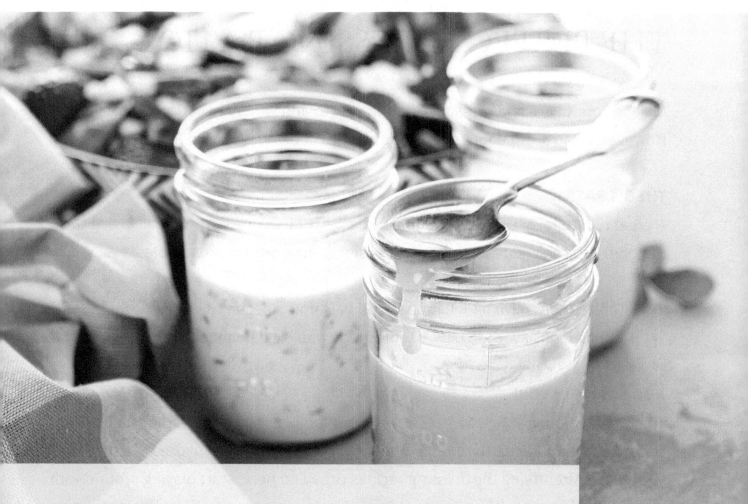

CHAPTER 6
DRESSINGS

THE PERFECT DRESSING RATIO

Making your own salad dressings is a fun way to add variety to your daily salads. However, it can seem daunting to find the perfect blend of oil, vinegar, and spices.

THE 3:1 RATIO

A great rule to follow is the 3:1 ratio... three parts oil to one part vinegar. Using this method, you can create lots of basic dressings. Here are a few examples:

- 3 Tablespoons olive oil + 1 Tablespoon balsamic vinegar
- 3 Tablespoons avocado oil + 1 Tablespoon apple cider vinegar

ADD SOME FLAVOR!

The fun of creating your own dressings is you can play around with different combinations of spices, herbs, oils, and acids to create a flavorful dressing that fits your taste. After trying the dressing recipes provided here, start playing around with different flavor combos!

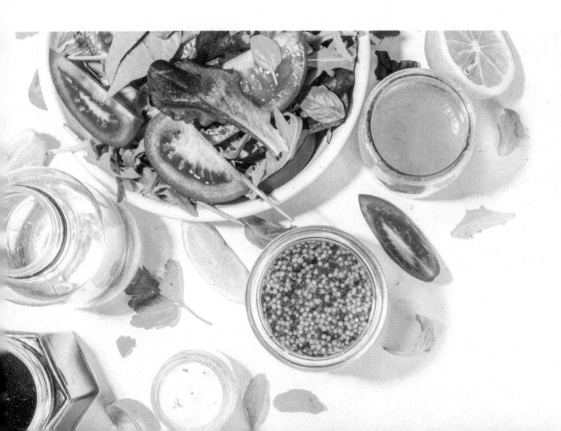

GO-TO SALAD DRESSINGS

BASIC VINAIGRETTE

- 3 Tablespoons olive oil + 1 Tablespoon balsamic vinegar + additions
- 3 Tablespoons avocado oil + 1 Tablespoon apple cider vinegar + additions

1 serving = 1 Tablespoon

Makes 9 servings

Calories: 65 | Total Fat: 6 g | Total Carb: 3 g | Protein: 0 g

FRESH BASIL VINAIGRETTE

- ½ cup fresh basil leaves
- 3 Tablespoons white balsamic vinegar
- 2 Tablespoons olive or avocado oil
- 2 Tablespoons water
- 1 Tablespoon honey
- 1 Tablespoon minced fresh garlic
- ½ teaspoon salt
- ½ teaspoon black pepper

1 serving = 1 Tablespoon

Makes 9 servings

Calories: Calories: 41 | Total Fat: 3 g | Total Carb: 3 g | Protein: 0 g

MAPLE BALSAMIC VINAIGRETTE

- ¼ cup olive oil
- ¼ cup balsamic vinegar
- ¼ cup maple syrup
- ½ - 1 teaspoon cinnamon
- ¼ teaspoon salt

This dressing is heavenly on an arugula salad with roasted sweet potato, onion, feta cheese, and chopped pecans.

1 serving = 1 Tablespoon

Makes 12 servings

Calories: 64 | Total Fat: 5 g | Total Carb: 5 g | Protein: 0 g

STRAWBERRY VINAIGRETTE

- ½ cup fresh strawberries
- 1 Tablespoon apple cider or white vinegar
- 2 Tablespoons olive oil
- ¼ teaspoon salt
- ¼ teaspoon pepper

1 serving = 1 Tablespoon

Makes 11 servings

Calories: 24 | Total Fat: 2 g | Total Carb: 1 g | Protein: 0 g

AVOCADO DRESSING

- ½ - 1 cup olive oil, depending on desired consistency
- ⅓ cup apple cider vinegar
- 1 Tablespoon lemon juice
- 1 avocado
- 1 Tablespoon whole-grain mustard
- 1 Tablespoon honey
- 1 Tablespoon fresh minced garlic
- Fresh basil and parsley, to taste
- ¼ teaspoon salt
- ¼ teaspoon pepper

1 serving = 1 Tablespoon

Makes 20 servings

Calories: 65 | Total Fat: 7 g | Total Carb: 2 g | Protein: 0 g

LEMON HERB VINAIGRETTE

- 6 Tablespoons olive oil
- 1 Tablespoon red wine or white vinegar
- 1 Tablespoon lemon juice
- 1 teaspoon oregano, fresh or dried
- 1 teaspoon basil, fresh or dried
- ½ teaspoon salt
- ½ teaspoon pepper

1 serving = 1 Tablespoon

Makes 9 servings

Calories: 80 | Total Fat: 9 g | Total Carb: 0 g | Protein: 0 g

PEANUT DRESSING

- 5 Tablespoons natural creamy peanut butter
- 2 Tablespoons coconut aminos or tamari (gluten-free soy sauce)
- 1 Tablespoon honey
- 3 Tablespoons water
- 1 teaspoon minced fresh garlic
- 1 teaspoon grated fresh ginger

1 serving = 1 Tablespoon

Makes 11 servings

Calories: 50 | Total Fat: 4 g | Total Carb: 4 g | Protein: 2 g

WARM SPICED TAHINI DRESSING

- ⅓ cup natural tahini
- 2 Tablespoons maple syrup
- 1 Tablespoon white vinegar or apple cider vinegar
- ¼ teaspoon cinnamon
- ¼ teaspoon allspice
- 3 Tablespoons water

1 serving = 1 Tablespoon

Makes 12 servings

Calories: 45 | Total Fat: 3 g | Total Carb: 3 g | Protein: 1 g

CHAPTER 7
FILLING SALADS

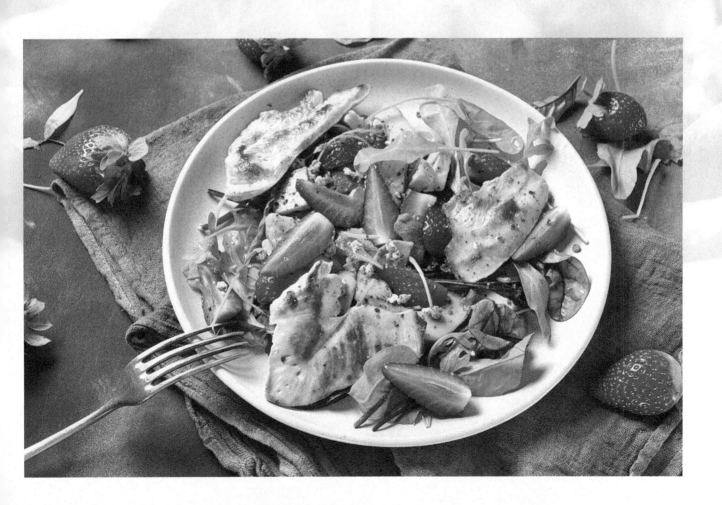

CHICKEN & PEACH ARUGULA SALAD

INGREDIENTS

- 2 cups baby arugula
- 4 chicken thighs, cooked and cut into bite-sized pieces
- 1 peach, cut into pieces
- ¼ red onion, sliced thinly
- 2 ounces of feta cheese crumbles
- ¼ cup chopped walnuts or pecans
- Fresh basil vinaigrette

DIRECTIONS

1. Cook the chicken thighs and cut them into bite-sized pieces.
2. Create a bed of arugula, then top with chicken, ½ a peach, 2 Tablespoons red onion, 1 ounce of feta cheese crumbles, and 2 Tablespoons chopped walnuts.
3. Drizzle basil vinaigrette over the salad and serve.

COOK TIME: 0 MIN
PREP TIME: 5 MIN
SERVINGS: 2

NUTRITION (not including dressing)

Calories: 337 | Total Fat: 24 g | Total Carb: 12 g | Protein: 21 g

GREEK CHICKEN SALAD

INGREDIENTS

- 1 head of lettuce, shredded or cut into wedges.
- ½ cup cucumber, diced
- ½ cup red bell peppers, diced
- ½ cup red onion, sliced thinly
- ½ cup cherry tomatoes, cut in half
- ½ cup kalamata olives, pitted
- 1 avocado, sliced
- 4 chicken breasts, cooked and cut into pieces
- 2 teaspoons dried oregano
- 2 teaspoons dried basil
- 2 teaspoons garlic powder
- salt and pepper to taste
- 4 ounces of feta cheese
- Your choice of dressing

DIRECTIONS

1. Cook the chicken breasts and cut them into pieces.
2. In a large bowl, combine the remaining salad ingredients and mix them together.
3. Top with your choice of dressing (see notes.)

NOTES

Several dressings would go well with this salad. Give them all a try and see which you prefer! My recommendation is to pair this salad with one of the following from our dressings section:

- basic vinaigrette
- fresh basil vinaigrette
- lemon herb vinaigrette

COOK TIME: 0 MIN
PREP TIME: 5 MIN
SERVINGS: 6

NUTRITION (not including dressing)

Calories: 282 | Total Fat: 17 g | Total Carb: 8 g | Protein: 21 g

MEDITERRANEAN TUNA SALAD

INGREDIENTS

- 3 cans tuna (12 ounces total, canned in water), drained
- 1 tomato, cut into small pieces
- 1 red bell pepper, diced
- ½ red onion, cut into small pieces
- 1 cucumber, cut into coins then halved, then halved (about 1 cup)
- 2 garlic cloves, minced (about 2 teaspoons)
- ½ cup canned chickpeas, drained and rinsed
- ½ cup kalamata olives
- ½ cup feta cheese crumbles
- ¼ cup fresh parsley, chopped
- Salt and pepper to taste
- 2 Tablespoons olive oil
- 1 Tablespoon lemon juice

DIRECTIONS

1. In a large bowl, combine all ingredients and mix until evenly distributed.
2. Serve immediately or store in the fridge for later.

COOK TIME: 0 MIN
PREP TIME: 10 MIN
SERVINGS: 4

NUTRITION

Calories: 298 | Total Fat: 17 g | Total Carb: 13 g | Protein: 24 g

BLACKBERRY WALNUT CHICKEN SALAD

INGREDIENTS

- 2 cups mixed greens, baby arugula, or baby spinach
- 2 turkey breasts (4 ounces each), cooked and sliced
- 1 cup blackberries
- ¼ cup walnuts
- 2 oz. goat cheese (optional)
- Basic vinaigrette

COOK TIME: 0 MIN
PREP TIME: 5 MIN
SERVINGS: 2

DIRECTIONS

1. Cook the turkey breasts and cut them into slices.
2. Create a bed of greens, then top it with turkey, blackberries, walnuts, and goat cheese.
3. Drizzle basic vinaigrette over the salad and serve.

NUTRITION (not including dressing)

Calories: 301 | Total Fat: 14 g | Total Carb: 11 g | Protein: 35 g

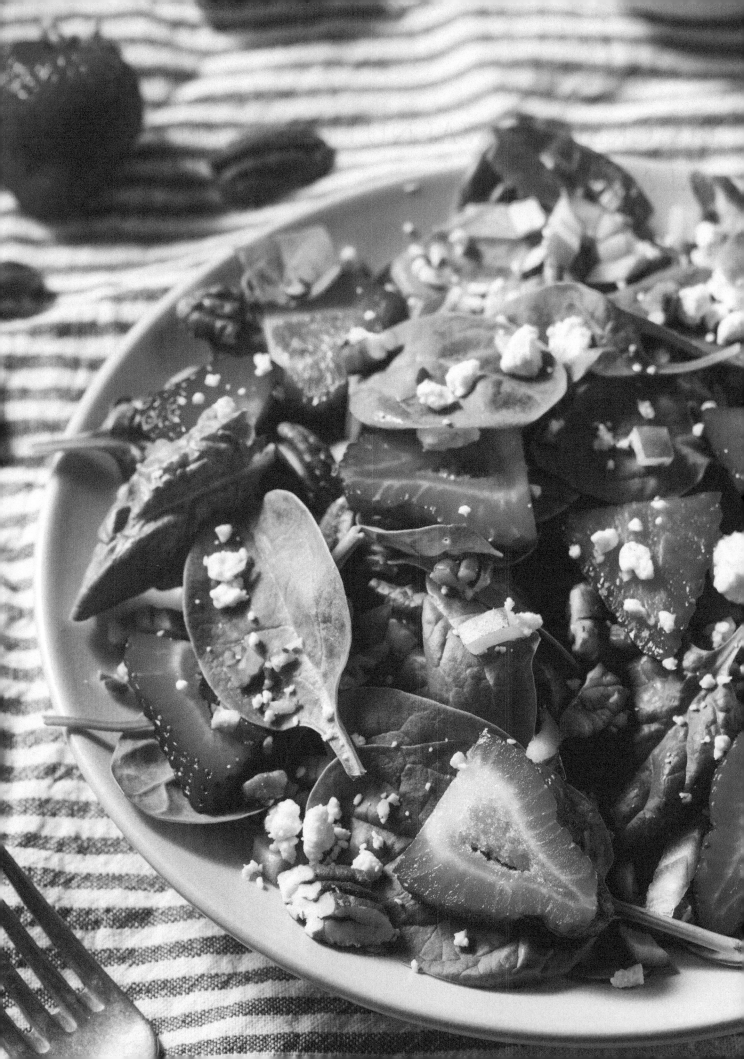

STRAWBERRY PECAN CHICKEN SALAD

INGREDIENTS

- 2 cups baby spinach
- 2 chicken breasts (4 oz. each), cooked and sliced
- 1 cup strawberries, halved or sliced
- ¼ cup red onion, chopped
- ¼ cup pecans, chopped
- 2 ounces feta cheese (optional)
- Fresh basil vinaigrette

COOK TIME: 0 MIN
PREP TIME: 5 MIN
SERVINGS: 2

DIRECTIONS

1. Cook the chicken breasts and cut them into slices.
2. Create a bed of baby spinach, then top it with chicken, strawberries, pecans, and feta cheese.
3. Drizzle basil vinaigrette over the salad and serve.

NUTRITION (not including dressing)

Calories: 360 | Total Fat: 15 g | Total Carb: 9 g | Protein: 43 g

BEEF, GUACAMOLE & HERBED GOAT CHEESE SALAD

INGREDIENTS

- 2 Tablespoons olive oil
- 1 pound ground beef (about 85% lean)
- 6 cups chopped romaine lettuce
- 1 cup cherry tomatoes, halved
- 4 ounces garlic herb goat cheese crumbled (I like the Taste of Inspiration brand)
- ¾ cup guacamole (or 3 Tablespoons per serving)

COOK TIME: 10 MIN
PREP TIME: 5 MIN
SERVINGS: 4

DIRECTIONS

1. Add the olive oil to a medium-sized saucepan.
2. Form the ground beef into small balls and cook over medium heat until cooked through (about 7-10 minutes). Once cooked, remove from heat.
3. Assemble the salads by dividing the lettuce, cherry tomatoes, and herbed goat cheese into four bowls.
4. Add the beef to each salad, top with roughly 3 Tablespoons of guacamole, and serve.

NOTES

- In this recipe, the guacamole serves as the dressing.

NUTRITION

Calories: 493 | Total Fat: 29 g | Total Carb: 5 g | Protein: 29 g

ROASTED BEET & BUTTERNUT SQUASH SALAD

INGREDIENTS

- 1 small butternut squash: peeled, cut in half, seeds scooped out, then chopped
- 3 whole beets
- Olive oil
- 4 ounces goat cheese
- 1 bunch fresh basil, chopped

COOK TIME: 60 MIN
PREP TIME: 10 MIN
SERVINGS: 6

NUTRITION

Calories: 150 | Total Fat: 4 g
Total Carb: 25 g | Protein: 5 g

DIRECTIONS

1. Preheat the oven to 425 degrees F.
2. Prepare the butternut squash by peeling it, cutting it in half, scooping the seeds out with a spoon, and cutting it into bite-sized pieces.
3. Put the butternut squash in a bowl, coat it with olive oil, and mix until evenly covered.
4. Place on a sheet pan in a single layer.
5. Prepare the beets by washing them, poking holes in them with a fork, then covering them with foil (similar to when baking whole potatoes).
6. Place on the sheet pan with the butternut squash or in their own 8x8 baking dish.
7. Bake the butternut squash for 20-25 minutes, until the squash is soft.
8. Bake the whole beets in the oven for 60 minutes or until a fork pokes easily into the beet. Remove from the oven once cooked.
9. Allow the beets to cool, then peel the skin and cut them into bite-sized pieces.
10. In a large bowl, combine the butternut squash and beets. Top with goat cheese and fresh basil and serve. This salad can be served warm or cold.

ROASTED SWEET POTATO & ONION SALAD

INGREDIENTS

- 2 cups baby arugula
- 1 medium sweet potato, diced
- 1 red onion, diced
- Salt and pepper
- 2 ounces goat cheese
- ¼ cup chopped pecans
- 4 Tablespoons fresh basil vinaigrette

COOK TIME: 25 MIN
PREP TIME: 5 MIN
SERVINGS: 2

NUTRITION (not including dressing)

Calories: 301 | Total Fat: 14 g | Total Carb: 11 g | Protein: 35 g

DIRECTIONS

1. Preheat the oven to 425 degrees.
2. In a bowl, mix the diced sweet potato and red onion with olive oil until evenly coated.
3. Place in a single layer on a greased sheet pan and season with salt and pepper.
4. Bake for 20-25 minutes, until the sweet potato and onion are soft.

Prepare your salad (makes 2 salads)

1. Place 1 cup of baby arugula in a bowl.
2. Add the roasted sweet potato and onion, 1 ounce goat cheese, 2 Tablespoons chopped pecans, and 2 Tablespoons basil vinaigrette.

NOTES

This recipe is a great meal prep option as the roasted sweet potato and onion keep well in the fridge for several days. Feel free to add protein such as chicken or salmon to this recipe to make a filling meal.

SALMON & ROASTED BROCCOLI SALAD

INGREDIENTS

- 8 ounce salmon fillet
- 2 cups fresh or frozen broccoli florets
- ½ red onion, sliced thinly
- 2 Tablespoons olive oil
- Salt and pepper to taste
- 2 cups arugula
- 4 Tablespoons chopped walnuts
- 4 Tablespoons dressing of choice (I recommend the avocado dressing, basil vinaigrette, or peanut dressing.)

COOK TIME: 25 MIN
PREP TIME: 5 MIN
SERVINGS: 2

NUTRITION (not including dressing)

Calories: 400 | Total Fat: 29 g
Total Carb: 6 g | Protein: 26 g

DIRECTIONS

1. Preheat the oven to 425 degrees.
2. Place the salmon in a small glass dish (greased) or on a small, greased baking sheet. Season with salt and pepper.
3. On a separate greased baking sheet, lay out the broccoli and onion in a single layer and drizzle olive oil on top. Season with salt and pepper.
4. Bake the salmon in the oven for 15-17 minutes, until the internal temperature is 145 degrees. Check after 15 minutes as it cooks quickly.
5. Roast the broccoli and onion in the oven for 15-25 minutes, until the florets are soft and crispy. Remove from the oven and allow to cool for several minutes.

Prepare your salad (makes 2 salads)

1. Place 1 cup of baby arugula in each bowl.
2. Add the salmon, roasted broccoli, roasted onion, and 2 Tablespoons of chopped walnuts to each bowl.
3. Dressing with 2 Tablespoons of your choice in dressing, and enjoy!

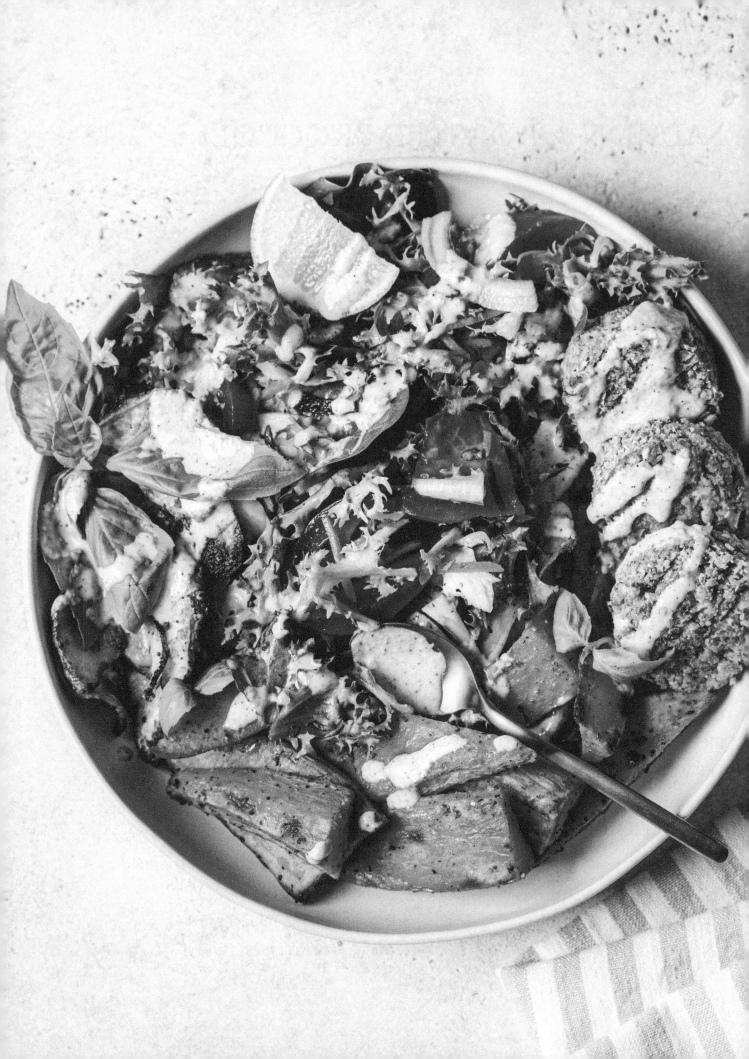

BUILD YOUR OWN SALAD BOWLS

CHOOSE YOUR BASE

There are so many options to choose from! My favorite "green" bases are arugula, baby spinach, and kale. They are nutritional superfoods and pair well with nearly any topping you choose.

CHOOSE YOUR VEGGIES

Play around with a variety of vegetable combinations to see what you prefer. You will eventually have your go-to favorites. My faves include sweet potato, red onion, mushrooms, eggplant, zucchini, and cherry tomatoes.

CHOOSE YOUR PROTEIN

A well-rounded salad is not complete without protein to keep you full for hours. This can be a meat protein such as chicken, turkey, or tuna, a plant protein such as quinoa or beans, or hard-boiled eggs.

CHOOSE YOUR DRESSING

Trying different dressings with different veggies is also fun to explore. Give our dressings here a try and find your favorite combinations.

FUN ADDITIONS

Lastly, add in some additions such as chopped nuts (walnuts, pecans, almonds, etc.), pumpkin seeds, dried cranberries, fresh berries, olives, feta cheese, goat cheese, fresh herbs, etc.

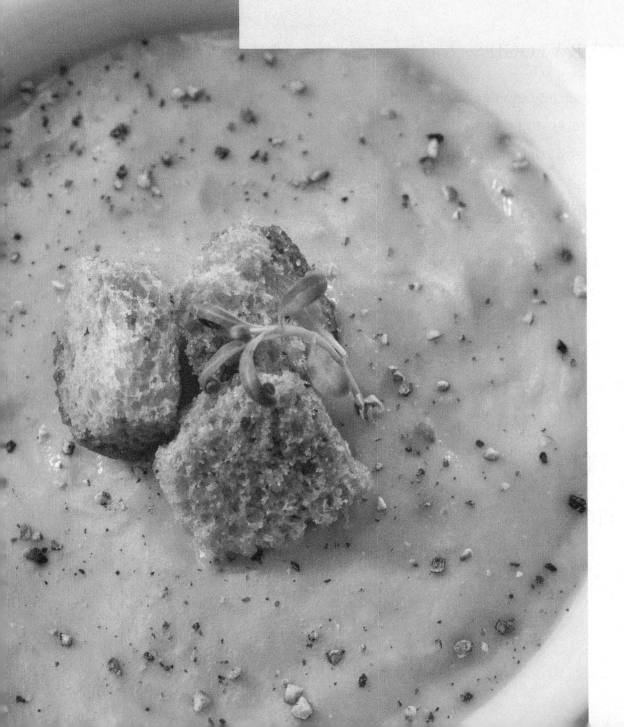

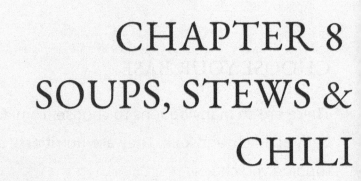

CHAPTER 8
SOUPS, STEWS &
CHILI

COMFORTING CHICKEN SOUP

INGREDIENTS

- 4 skinless, boneless chicken thighs
- 2 Tablespoons olive oil
- 5 medium-sized carrots, sliced
- 5 stalks of celery, sliced
- 1 yellow onion, diced
- 2 teaspoons salt
- 2 teaspoons pepper
- 2 teaspoons Italian seasoning
- 8 cups chicken broth

COOK TIME: 30 MIN
PREP TIME: 10 MIN
SERVINGS: 8

NUTRITION

Calories: 173 | Total Fat: 6 g
Total Carb: 6 g | Protein: 17 g

DIRECTIONS

1. In a large pot, add the olive oil and chicken thighs and cook over medium heat.
2. Cook the chicken thighs for 3 minutes, then flip the thighs and cook for an additional 3 minutes, until the chicken is fully cooked through.
3. Add 1 cup of the chicken broth to the pot, then cover the pot with a lid and allow the chicken to cook for 10 more minutes until completely cooked through.
4. Remove the chicken from the pot, shred it with a fork, and set it to the side.
5. Add the carrots, celery, onion, salt, pepper, Italian seasoning, and remaining chicken broth to the pot and bring to a boil.
6. Once boiling, reduce the heat and allow the soup to simmer for 15 minutes.
7. Once the vegetables are soft, add the shredded chicken, mix them together, then serve.

CHICKEN SAUSAGE & KALE SOUP

INGREDIENTS

- 2 Tablespoons olive oil
- 1 yellow onion, diced
- 3 garlic cloves, minced
- Salt and pepper
- 3 red potatoes, cut into bite-sized pieces
- 6 cups chicken stock
- 2 cups fresh kale
- 4 Italian chicken sausages, sliced

COOK TIME: 20 MIN
PREP TIME: 10 MIN
SERVINGS: 4

NUTRITION

Calories: 273 | Total Fat: 10 g | Total Carb: 28 g | Protein: 19 g

DIRECTIONS

1. In a medium-large pot, add olive oil, diced onion, garlic cloves, salt, and pepper, and cook over medium heat. Allow the diced onion to cook and become soft.
2. Add the potatoes and chicken stock and bring to a simmer. Allow to simmer for about 20 minutes or until the potatoes are soft and you can easily poke through with a fork.
3. Add the kale and allow them to soften.
4. Cook for 5-10 more minutes, then add the chicken sausage and allow to heat through.
5. Serve immediately or enjoy later.

NOTES

This soup freezes well and can be easily reheated for on-the-go lunches or last-minute meals.

TURKEY CHILI

INGREDIENTS

- 1 pound ground turkey
- 1 Tablespoon minced garlic
- 1 yellow onion, diced
- 1 (15-ounce) can diced tomatoes, drained
- 1 (15-ounce) can tomato sauce
- 1 (7-ounce) can diced green chiles
- 1 (4-ounce) can diced jalapeños
- 1 (15-ounce) can kidney beans, drained and rinsed
- 1 (15-ounce) can black beans, drained and rinsed
- 2 Tablespoons chili powder
- 2 teaspoons cumin
- 2 teaspoons garlic powder
- ½ teaspoon salt
- ½ teaspoon pepper

COOK TIME: 15 MIN
PREP TIME: 5 MIN
SERVINGS: 5

NUTRITION

Calories: 374 | Total Fat: 8 g | Total Carb: 45 g Protein: 31 g

DIRECTIONS

1. In a large pot, brown the turkey over medium heat. Add the garlic and diced onion to allow to cook with the turkey.
2. Once the turkey is cooked, add the remaining ingredients to the pot and bring to a simmer.
3. Allow to simmer for about 10 minutes, then serve.

NOTES

- Add chopped scallions or a few tablespoons of high-quality shredded cheese for a delicious, high-protein meal.
- Make sure to rinse canned beans before adding them to the chili. Dump beans into a colander and rinse until there are no more "bubbles" in the beans. These bubbles are what can cause gas and bloating after consumption.

LENTIL SOUP (WITH INSTANT POT & STOVETOP DIRECTIONS)

INGREDIENTS

- 1½ cups French green lentils, dry (use 1½ - 15 ounce cans if making stovetop version)
- 4 cloves garlic, minced
- 1 (15-ounce) can fire roasted diced tomatoes
- 1 (15-ounce) can crushed tomatoes
- 4 cups chicken or vegetable broth
- 2 Tablespoons olive oil
- 1 yellow onion, diced
- 4 medium carrots, diced
- 4 celery stalks, diced
- 4 sprigs of fresh thyme, whole
- 1 teaspoon salt
- 1 teaspoon smoked paprika

COOK TIME: 20 MIN
PREP TIME: 5 MIN
SERVINGS: 6

DIRECTIONS

Instant Pot Directions:
1. Add all of the ingredients to the instant pot and stir until everything is combined.
2. Put on the lid of the Instant Pot and seal.
3. Cook on high pressure for 15 minutes. Once the Instant Pot is done, allow the pressure to naturally release.
4. Open the lid and remove the thyme sprigs.
5. Stir the soup, add additional salt and pepper if you'd prefer, then serve.

Stovetop Directions:
1. Replace the dried lentils with 1½ (15-ounce) cans of lentils
2. Add all of the ingredients to a large pot and simmer for 15-20 minutes.

NUTRITION

Calories: 279 | Total Fat: 35 g
Total Carb: 46 g | Protein: 13 g

WHITE BEAN & BACON SOUP

INGREDIENTS

- ½ pound thick-cut bacon, cooked and cut into pieces
- 2 (14.5-ounce) cans cannellini or great northern beans, drained and rinsed
- 1 cup carrots, chopped
- 4 cups chicken broth
- 1 Tablespoon minced garlic
- Salt and pepper to taste
- Rosemary to garnish

COOK TIME: 20 MIN
PREP TIME: 5 MIN
SERVINGS: 6

NUTRITION

Calories: 380 | Total Fat: 14 g | Total Carb: 33 g | Protein: 27 g

DIRECTIONS

1. Cook the bacon, allow it to cool enough to handle, then tear it into pieces.
2. In a large pot, combine the bacon, cannellini beans, carrots, chicken broth, garlic, salt, and pepper. Bring to a simmer over medium heat and allow to simmer until the carrots become soft (about 20 minutes).
3. Serve warm, garnished with fresh rosemary.

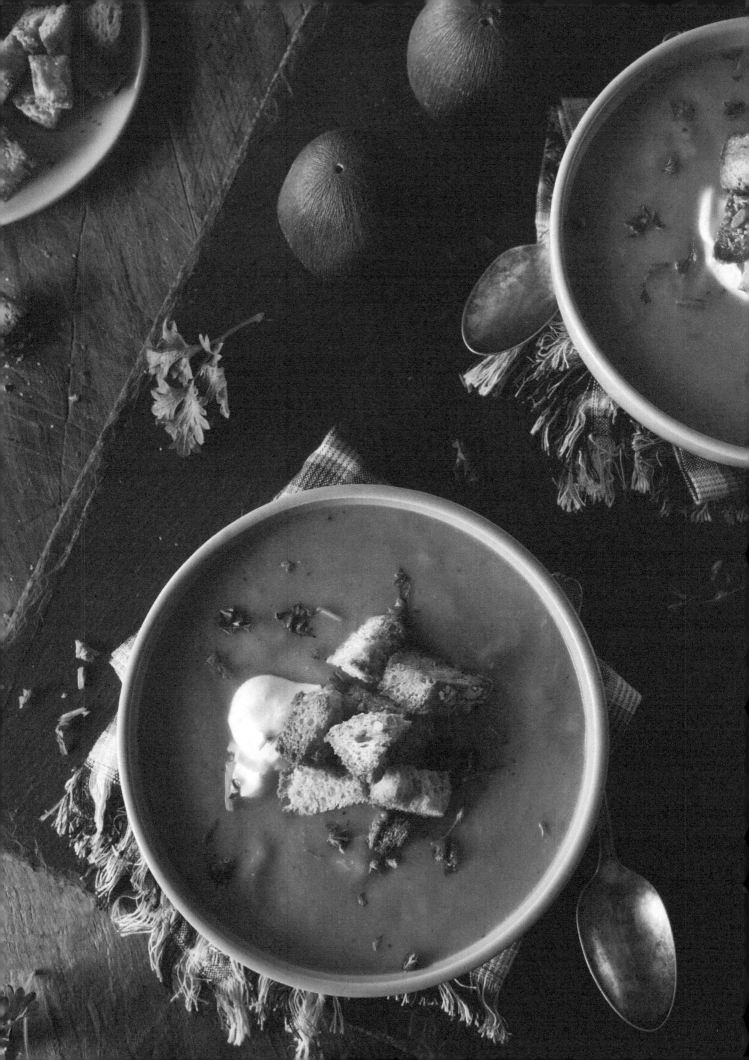

ROASTED BUTTERNUT SQUASH SOUP

INGREDIENTS

- 4 cups diced butternut squash
- 1 small red onion, diced
- 2 Tablespoons avocado oil
- ½ teaspoon salt
- ½ teaspoon ground black pepper
- 2½ cups chicken broth
- 4 garlic cloves, minced
- ½ teaspoon dried sage
- ¼ teaspoon cinnamon
- ⅛ teaspoon nutmeg
- 1 ½ Tablespoons nutritional yeast

Optional garnishes:
- Nitrate-free bacon, cooked and crumbled
- Diced green onion
- Pumpkin seeds

COOK TIME: 40 MIN
PREP TIME: 10 MIN
SERVINGS: 6

DIRECTIONS

1. Preheat the oven to 425 degrees F.
2. Spread the diced butternut squash and red onion on a sheet pan lined with parchment paper. Drizzle with avocado oil and mix up until the squash is evenly coated with oil. Sprinkle salt and pepper over the veggies.
3. Roast in a preheated oven for 30 minutes, mixing up halfway through for even roasting.
4. Remove the squash and onion from the oven and allow them cool for a few minutes. Then, transfer the squash to a blender or food processor.
5. Add the chicken broth, applesauce, minced garlic, sage, cinnamon, nutmeg, and nutritional yeast to the blender. **Remove the heat release cap and loosely place a towel over it to prevent spills.** Blend until the mixture is smooth and creamy.
6. Transfer to a bowl, garnish as desired, and serve.

NUTRITION

Calories: 84 | Total Fat: 5 g | Total Carb: 9 g | Protein: 2 g

ROASTED CAULIFLOWER & BROCCOLI SOUP

INGREDIENTS

- 2 cups broccoli florets (fresh or frozen)
- 2 cups cauliflower florets (fresh or frozen)
- 2 Tablespoons olive oil
- salt and pepper to taste
- 2 cloves garlic, minced (about 2 teaspoons)
- 1 cup unsweetened almond milk or coconut milk
- Optional garnishes: crumbled bacon, freshly shredded parmesan

COOK TIME: 25 MIN
PREP TIME: 5 MIN
SERVINGS: 4

NUTRITION

Calories: 95 | Total Fat: 7 g | Total Carb: 4 g | Protein: 2 g

DIRECTIONS

1. Preheat the oven to 425 degrees F.
2. In a bowl, add the broccoli and cauliflower. Drizzle the olive oil over the veggies and mix until evenly covered.
3. Dump the veggies onto a greased baking sheet and spread them so they are in a single layer. Season with salt and pepper.
4. Bake for 20-25 minutes, until the broccoli and cauliflower are crispy.
5. Remove from the oven, then using a spatula, put the veggies in a blender or food processor.
6. Add the minced garlic and almond milk to the blender.
7. **Make sure to remove the vent piece from the blender's lid before turning on the blender. When blending hot ingredients, you must allow it to vent or the pressure will build up from the hot food. Place a towel over the open area to prevent it from splashing out.**
8. Blend to desired consistency, and add more milk if you would like the soup to be thicker.
9. Add additional garnishes to the soup after pouring the soup into serving bowls.

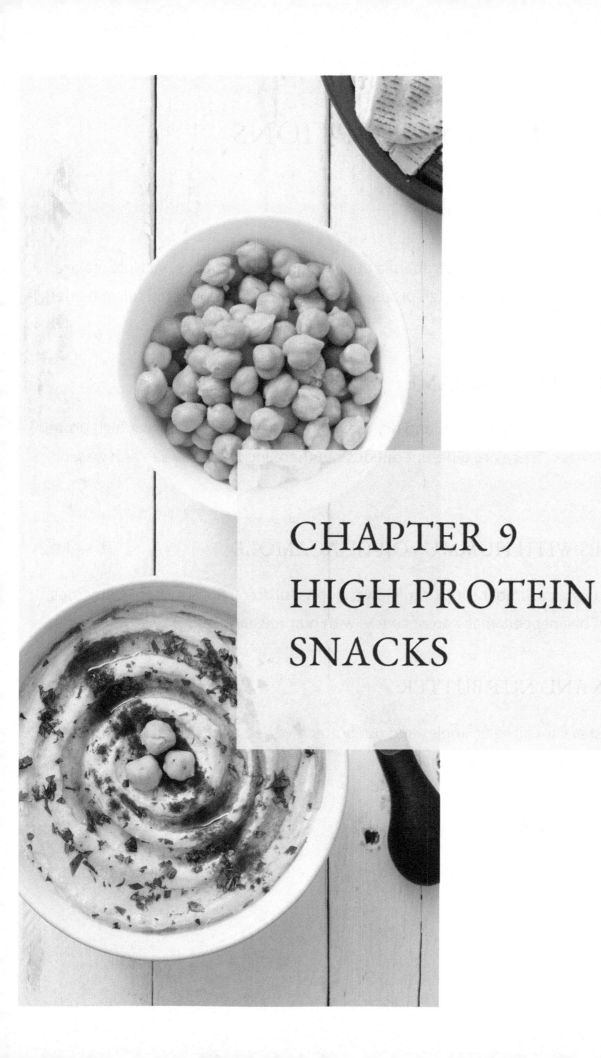

CHAPTER 9
HIGH PROTEIN
SNACKS

HEALTHY SNACK OPTIONS

NUTS

Cashews, almonds, pecans, macadamia nuts, walnuts, the list goes on! Nuts make a great snack option with their high protein and fat content, keeping you full and energy-filled for hours.

DRY ROASTED EDAMAME

Edamame are whole soy beans, and dry roasted edamame makes a great high protein, high fiber snack. There are different options out there including sea salt and wasabi flavored.

VEGGIES WITH HUMMUS OR GUACAMOLE

Carrots, celery, cucumber slices, cauliflower florets, broccoli florets, cherry tomatoes, and sliced bell peppers make great snacks with hummus and guacamole.

APPLES AND NUT BUTTER

A classic snack for all ages, apples and nut butter give you a little bit of sweetness and a whole lot of fiber and healthy fat.

GREEK YOGURT

Greek yogurt is high in protein and makes a delicious, filling snack when combined with berries and nuts.

PERFECT DEVILED EGGS

INGREDIENTS

- ¼ cup baking soda
- 6 eggs
- 1 teaspoon yellow mustard
- ¼ cup mayonnaise made with olive or avocado oil (or use Greek yogurt)
- Smoked paprika
- Salt & pepper, to taste

COOK TIME: 15 MIN
PREP TIME: 5 MIN
SERVINGS: 6

NUTRITION

Calories: 112 | Total Fat: 9 g
Total Carb: 1 g | Protein: 6 g

DIRECTIONS

1. Fill a large pot with water and add ¼ cup of baking soda to the water. This makes the egg shells come off a lot easier for peeling.
2. Add the eggs to the pot.
3. Set the stove on high and bring it to a boil.
4. Once boiling, set your timer to 10 minutes.
5. After 10 minutes, allow the eggs to cool in the pot with the water or move the eggs to a bowl of ice water, which can also aid in peeling the shells off more easily.
6. Once cooled, peel off the egg shells and cut the eggs in half.
7. Scoop out the yolks and add to a bowl.
8. Add the yellow mustard, mayonnaise, salt, and pepper to the bowl with the egg yolks.
9. Scoop the mixture back into the egg whites, then sprinkle with smoked paprika.

SPICED NUTS

INGREDIENTS

- 3 cups total of assorted **raw** nuts. Options include almonds, pecans, walnuts, cashews, Brazil nuts, hazelnuts, macadamia nuts, pistachios, etc.
- 1½ Tablespoons olive oil
- ½ teaspoon coarse pink Himalayan salt
- ½ teaspoon cumin
- ½ teaspoon chili powder
- ¼ teaspoon dried garlic
- ¼ teaspoon cayenne
- ⅛ teaspoon pepper

COOK TIME: 15 MIN
PREP TIME: 5 MIN
SERVINGS: 12

DIRECTIONS

1. Preheat the oven to 350 degrees F.
2. In a bowl, combine the nuts, olive oil, and spices. Mix until evenly coated.
3. Lay the nuts out into a baking sheet lined with parchment paper, making sure they are in a single layer.
4. Bake for 15 minutes, then remove from the oven.
5. Store in an airtight container once completely cooled.

NUTRITION (¼ cup)

Calories: 112 | Total Fat: 9 g
Total Carb: 1 g | Protein: 6 g

AVOCADO TOAST

INGREDIENTS

- 1 slice whole grain or gluten-free bread, toasted
- ½ avocado
- ½ teaspoon lemon juice
- Salt and pepper to taste
- Red pepper flakes to taste

COOK TIME: 0 MIN
PREP TIME: 5 MIN
SERVINGS: 1

NUTRITION

Calories: 210 | Total Fat: 12 g
Total Carb: 22 g | Protein: 4 g

DIRECTIONS

1. Toast a piece of your favorite whole grain or gluten free bread.
2. Cut an avocado in half and remove the pit.
3. Using a knife, cut the avocado into chunks while still in the peel.
4. Use a spoon to scoop out the avocado and add it to a bowl. Add the lemon juice to the bowl.
5. Use a fork to slightly mash up the avocado, then spread the mashed avocado onto the toasted bread.
6. Season with salt, pepper, and red pepper flake to taste, then enjoy!

PEANUT BUTTER, RAISIN & COCONUT TOAST

INGREDIENTS

- 1 slice whole grain or gluten-free toast
- 1 Tablespoon natural peanut butter
- 2 Tablespoons shredded unsweetened coconut
- 1 Tablespoon raisins

DIRECTIONS

1. Toast a piece of your favorite whole grain or gluten free bread.
2. Spread all-natural peanut butter onto the toast, then sprinkle shredded coconut on top.
3. Add 1 Tablespoon raisin to the toast for a pop of sweetness.

COOK TIME: 15 MIN
PREP TIME: 5 MIN
SERVINGS: 1

NUTRITION

Calories: 290 | Total Fat: 16 g | Total Carb: 30 g | Protein: 7 g

ROASTED PEARS WITH HONEY & GREEK YOGURT

INGREDIENTS

- 2 pears
- 2 Tablespoons grass-fed butter or ghee, melted
- ½ teaspoon cinnamon
- 2 Tablespoons honey
- ½ - ¾ cup Greek Yogurt
- Optional addition: chopped walnuts or pecans

COOK TIME: 30 MIN
PREP TIME: 5 MIN
SERVINGS: 4

DIRECTIONS

1. Preheat the oven to 350 degrees F.
2. Grease an 8x8 baking dish and set aside.
3. Cut the pears in half and remove the cores.
4. Place the pears cut side up on a greased 8x8 baking dish.
5. Brush butter onto the pears and sprinkle with cinnamon.
6. Bake for 30 minutes, then remove from the oven.
7. Serve with 2-3 Tablespoons of Greek Yogurt, a drizzle of honey, and chopped walnuts or pecans.

NOTES

This recipe also works with peaches and apples and is a great way to enjoy fruit for a snack or dessert.

NUTRITION

Calories: 140 | Total Fat: 6 g | Total Carb: 23 g | Protein: 1 g

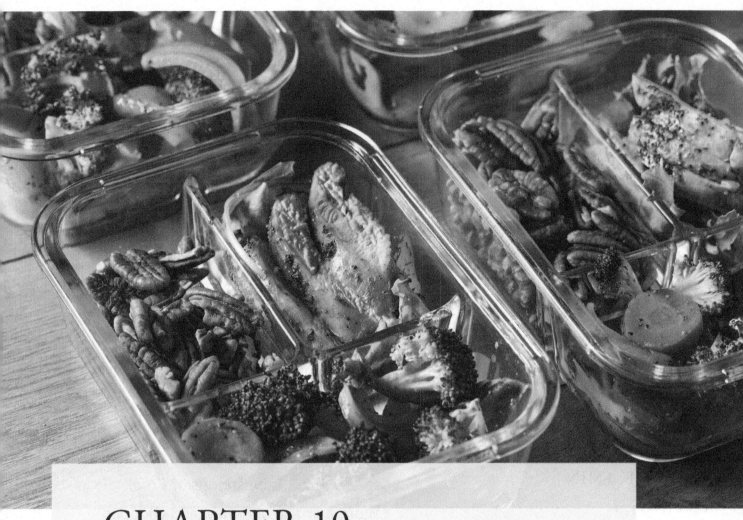

CHAPTER 10
MEAL PLANNING

GETTING STARTED

Now that we have reviewed an array of recipes to choose from, let's take a look at our meal plan!

This 30-day meal plan provides an outline of meals for breakfast, lunch, dinner, and snacks. This outline does not use leftovers as I understand not everyone is a fan. However, if you do enjoy leftovers and meal prepping, the next 30 days may be a little easier as you won't have to cook as much.

USING LEFTOVERS

If you are going to eat leftovers, my recommendation is to use the leftovers from dinner for the next day's lunch. You may not have leftovers each day, but this will give you an opportunity to incorporate some of the delicious salads that we often plan for lunches.

MEAL PLANNING VS. INTUITIVE EATING

This meal plan is just one example of the meals you might eat over the coming weeks. If you are more of an intuitive eater and prefer to plan meals day-by-day according to what you are craving (in a healthy way, of course), simply choose any of the meals in this guide, and you will still be on the right track toward a balanced, Mediterranean-based diet.

BE MINDFUL OF SNACKS

The following meal plan assumes that snacks will be consumed and, therefore, may not provide the total number of calories you need to consume each day with just the three meals outlined. Please be mindful of this and plan accordingly to ensure you are consuming the appropriate number of calories each day. Also, be mindful that some snacks are higher in calories than others. Nuts, for example, are generally higher in calories per serving than a piece of fruit.

ROASTED VEGETABLES

In the following meal plan, I simply list "roasted vegetables" to go with some of the meals. I do this to give you the opportunity to explore a variety of vegetables over the coming weeks and to discover your favorites.

TRACK YOUR PROGRESS WITH MYFITNESS PAL

Lastly, this is just a reminder that I highly recommend tracking your progress and calories consumed each day with MyFitness Pal or a similar program. This will ensure you are reaching your caloric goals each day and will provide support and accountability to give you the best chance of success in reaching your goals.

Let's get started!

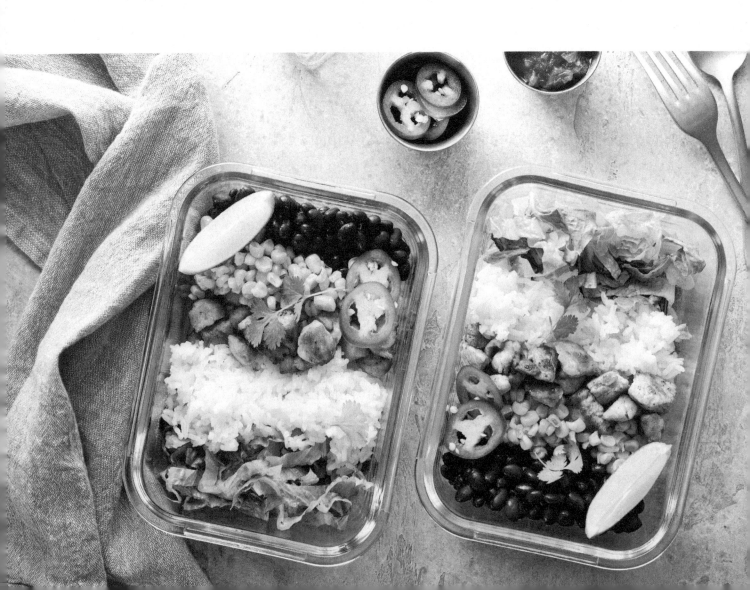

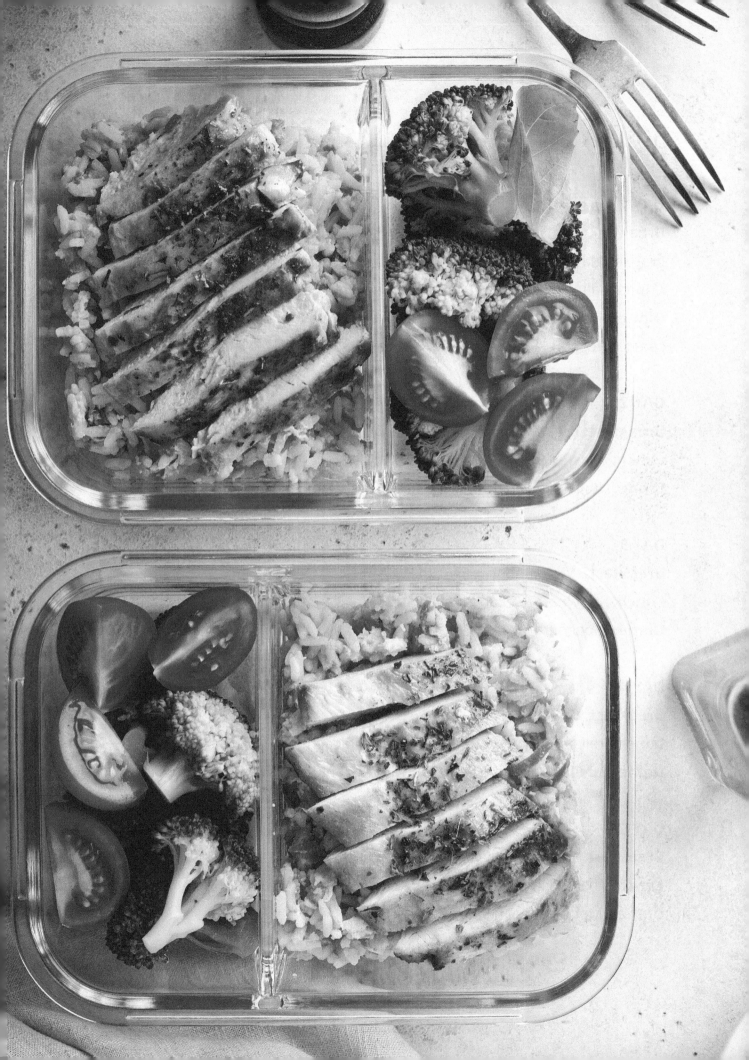

30 DAY MEAL PLAN

DAY 1

Breakfast: Mediterranean Scrambled Eggs, nitrate-free bacon, and a piece of whole-grain or gluten-free toast with grass-fed butter or ghee

Lunch: Salmon & Broccoli with Balsamic Reduction

Dinner: Mediterranean Pork Tenderloin with roasted potatoes and your choice of roasted vegetable

DAY 2

Breakfast: Eggs with Savory Pork Sausage Patties

Lunch: Roasted Sweet Potato & Onion Salad

Dinner: Italian Sausage with Zucchini, Feta & Quinoa

DAY 3

Breakfast: White Beans & Eggs in Purgatory

Lunch: Strawberry Pecan Chicken Salad

Dinner: Spaghetti Squash Chicken Marinara

DAY 4

Breakfast: Greek Feta Frittata

Lunch: Italian Chicken Patties with your choice of a roasted vegetable

Dinner: Mediterranean Baked Cod with Roasted Tomatoes and Artichoke

DAY 5

Breakfast: Easy Muesli with whole, plain Greek Yogurt and fresh berries

Lunch: Roasted Zucchini, Onion & Tomatoes with a side of quinoa

Dinner: Mediterranean Tuna Salad

DAY 6

Breakfast: Classic Frittata

Lunch: Greek Chicken Salad

Dinner: Sausage & Kale Soup

DAY 7

Breakfast: Chia Pudding with your choice of toppings

Lunch: Blackberry Walnut Turkey Salad with your choice of dressing

Dinner: Simple Beef Burger on a bed of lettuce, tomato, and red onion, topped with Primal Kitchen's Ketchup or BBQ sauce

DAY 8

Breakfast: Avocado Toast & Eggs

Lunch: Ground Beef Stir Fry

Dinner: Baked Trout with Loaded Mediterranean Potatoes

DAY 9

Breakfast: Easy Muesli with Greek yogurt and berries

Lunch: Roasted Eggplant, Zucchini, Mushroom & Red Onion Bowl

Dinner: Turkey breast with Apple & Pecan Stuffed Sweet Potatoes

DAY 10

Breakfast: Easy Banana Pancakes

Lunch: Baked Margherita Chicken

Dinner: Steak & Onions with a side salad

DAY 11

Breakfast: Mediterranean Breakfast Bowl

Lunch: Tuna Cakes with arugula, cherry tomatoes, sliced cucumber, and Avocado Dressing

Dinner: Baked chicken with your choice of roasted vegetable

DAY 12

Breakfast: Chia Pudding with your choice of toppings

Lunch: Bacon & Brussel Sprouts Slaw with baked chicken

Dinner: Margarita Flatbread with a side of roasted vegetables

DAY 13

Breakfast: Sweet Potato & Egg Skillet

Lunch: Greek Chicken Gyros with Tzatziki Sauce

Dinner: Classic Chicken Soup

DAY 14

Breakfast: Eggs with Low-Carb Waffles

Lunch: Roasted Beet & Butternut Squash Salad with chicken or turkey

Dinner: Greek Shrimp & Feta with a side of quinoa

DAY 15

Breakfast: Greek Feta Frittata

Lunch: Chicken & Peach Arugula Salad

Dinner: Turkey Chili

DAY 16

Breakfast: White Beans & Eggs in Purgatory

Lunch: Greek Chicken Salad

Dinner: Baked Turkey, Zucchini, Spinach & Feta Casserole

DAY 17

Breakfast: Classic Frittata

Lunch: Spaghetti Squash Chicken Marinara

Dinner: Mediterranean Pork Tenderloin with roasted potatoes and your choice of a second roasted vegetable

DAY 18

Breakfast: Chia Pudding with toppings of your choosing

Lunch: Ratatouille with a side of quinoa

Dinner: Mediterranean Baked Cod with Roasted Tomatoes and Artichoke

DAY 19

Breakfast: Mediterranean Scrambled Eggs, nitrate-free bacon, and whole-grain or gluten-free toast with grass-fed butter or ghee

Lunch: Beef, Guacamole & Herbed Goat Cheese Salad

Dinner: Sheet Pan Beef & Broccoli

DAY 20

Breakfast: Easy Muesli with whole, plain Greek Yogurt and fresh berries

Lunch: Roasted Butternut Squash Soup

Dinner: Salmon & Broccoli with Balsamic Reduction

DAY 21

Breakfast: Traditional Shakshuka

Lunch: Blackberry Walnut Turkey Salad with your choice of dressing

Dinner: Low-Carb Pizza Bowl

DAY 22

Breakfast: Eggs with Savory Pork Sausage Patties

Lunch: Lentil Soup

Dinner: Unstuffed Bell Peppers

DAY 23

Breakfast: Avocado Toast & Eggs

Lunch: Roasted Zucchini, Onion & Tomatoes with a side of quinoa

Dinner: Baked Margherita Chicken

DAY 24

Breakfast: White Beans & Eggs in Purgatory

Lunch: Mediterranean Tuna Salad

Dinner: Steak & Onions with a side salad

DAY 25

Breakfast: Classic Frittata

Lunch: Strawberry Pecan Chicken Salad

Dinner: Sausage & Kale Soup

DAY 26

Breakfast: Mediterranean Breakfast Bowl

Lunch: Salmon & Roasted Broccoli Salad

Dinner: Slow Cooker Spiced Pulled Pork with your choice of roasted vegetable

DAY 27

Breakfast: Easy Banana Pancakes

Lunch: Roasted Cauliflower & Broccoli Soup with chicken or turkey

Dinner: Greek Chicken Gyros with Tzatziki Sauce

DAY 28

Breakfast: Chia Pudding with your choice of toppings

Lunch: Bacon & Brussel Sprouts Slaw with baked chicken

Dinner: Baked Trout with Loaded Mediterranean Potatoes and your choice of roasted vegetable

DAY 29

Breakfast: Sweet Potato & Egg Skillet

Lunch: Chicken & Peach Arugula Salad

Dinner: Caramelized Onion & Spinach Flatbread

DAY 30

Breakfast: Mediterranean Scrambled Eggs

Lunch: Roasted Beet & Butternut Squash Salad

Dinner: Salmon & Broccoli with Balsamic Reduction

YOUR PERSONAL MEAL PLAN

	BREAKFAST	LUNCH	DINNER	SNACK
MON				
TUE				
WEN				
THU				
FRI				
SAT				
SUN				

YOUR PERSONAL MEAL PLAN

	BREAKFAST	LUNCH	DINNER	SNACK
MON				
TUE				
WEN				
THU				
FRI				
SAT				
SUN				

YOUR PERSONAL MEAL PLAN

	BREAKFAST	LUNCH	DINNER	SNACK
MON				
TUE				
WEN				
THU				
FRI				
SAT				
SUN				

YOUR PERSONAL MEAL PLAN

	BREAKFAST	LUNCH	DINNER	SNACK
MON				
TUE				
WEN				
THU				
FRI				
SAT				
SUN				

Helpful Articles from Beyond the Brambleberry

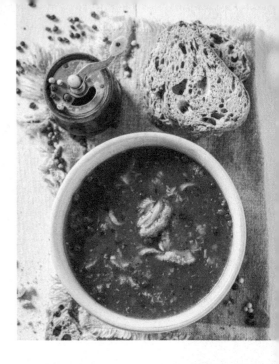

The following articles may be useful as you complete this 30-day meal plan. You can read the articles at **www.beyondthebrambleberry.com**.

How to Save Money on the Mediterranean Diet

The Top 5 Reasons You Aren't Losing Weight on the Mediterranean Diet (And How to Fix It)

How to Follow the Mediterranean Diet If You Hate Cooking or Have No Time

How to Manage Sugar Cravings on the Mediterranean Diet

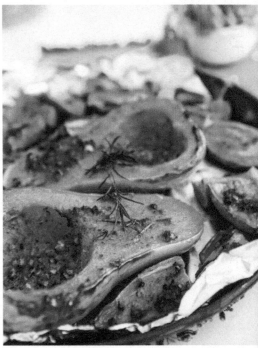

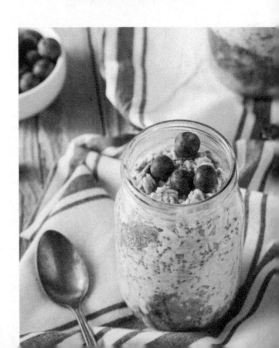

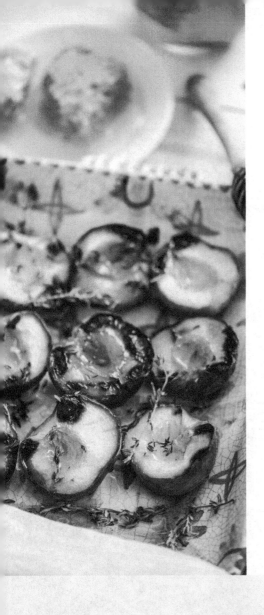

SHOP & RECOMMENDATIONS

I have put together a resource library containing my top recommended books, kitchen must-haves, supplements to support your health, and more. You can check it out at: https://www.beyondthebrambleberry.com/resource-page.

Connect with me

I would love to keep in touch and hear how you are enjoying these recipes. Connect with me via Instagram, Pinterest, or our weekly email newsletter.

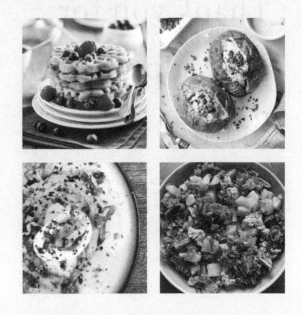

@beyondthebrambleberry

www.pinterest.com/beyondthebrambleberry/

Sign up for our weekly email newsletter at www.beyondthebrambleberry.com.

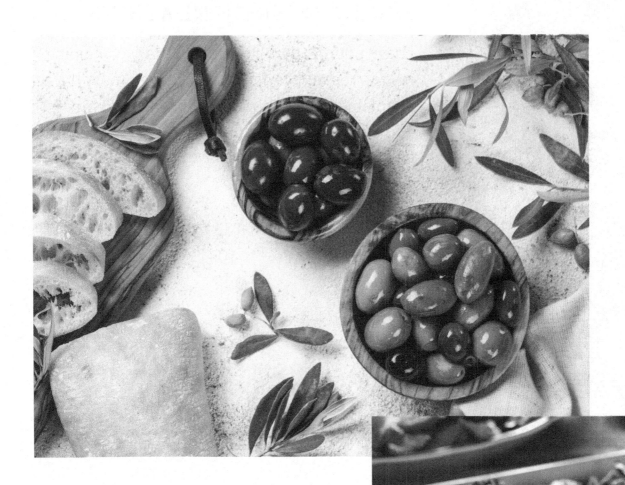

Thank you for
your support of
Beyond the
Brambleberry

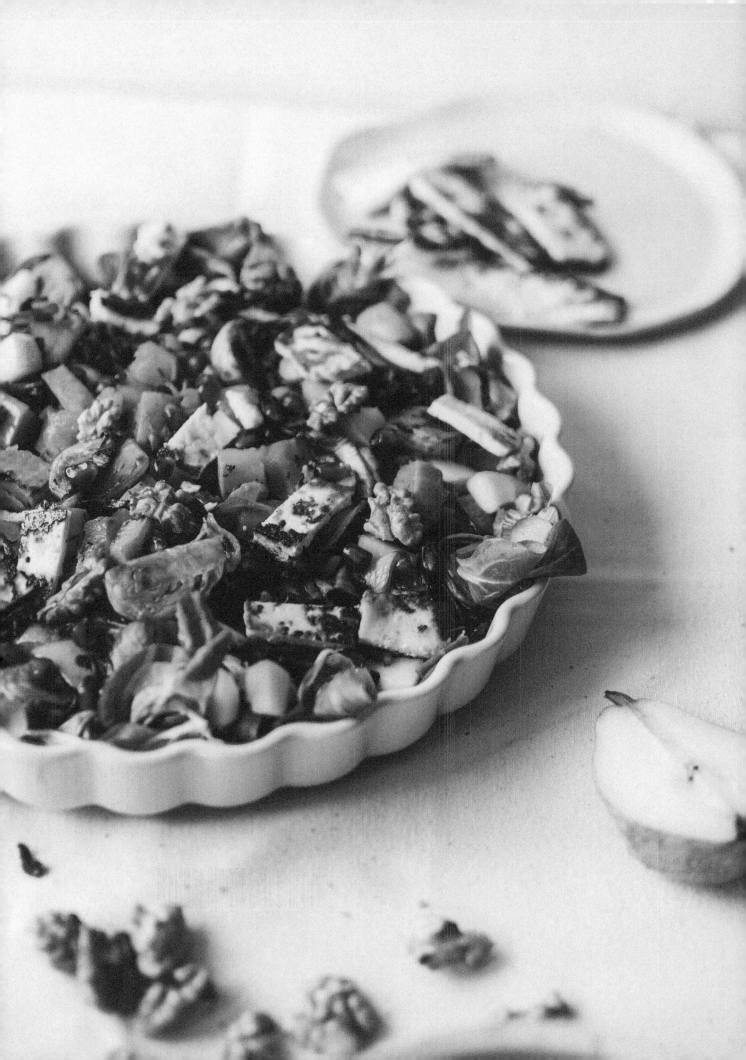

Made in the USA
Las Vegas, NV
28 January 2024

85038114R10090